D1392932

C... COMMISSIONING AND PUBLIC HEALTH

Linda Marks

LIS - LIBRARY

Date	Fund
27/6/17	nm -warr

Order No.	
283151x	

| University of Chester | |

First published in Great Britain in 2014 by

Policy Press
University of Bristol
6th Floor
Howard House
Queen's Avenue
Clifton
Bristol BS8 1SD
UK
t: +44 (0)117 331 5020
pp-info@bristol.ac.uk
www.policypress.co.uk

North America office:
Policy Press
c/o The University of Chicago Press
1427 East 60th Street
Chicago, IL 60637, USA
t: +1 773 702 7700
f: +1 773-702-9756
sales@press.uchicago.edu
www.press.uchicago.edu

© Policy Press 2014

British Library Cataloguing in Publication Data
A catalogue record for this book is available from the British Library

Library of Congress Cataloging-in-Publication Data
A catalog record for this book has been requested

ISBN 978 1 44730 493 7 paperback
ISBN 978 1 44730 494 4 hardcover

The right of Linda Marks to be identified as author of this work has been asserted by her in accordance with the Copyright, Designs and Patents Act 1988.

All rights reserved: no part of this publication may be reproduced, stored in a retrieval system, or transmitted in any form or by any means, electronic, mechanical, photocopying, recording, or otherwise without the prior permission of Policy Press.

The statements and opinions contained within this publication are solely those of the author and not of the University of Bristol or Policy Press. The University of Bristol and Policy Press disclaim responsibility for any injury to persons or property resulting from any material published in this publication.

Department of Health disclaimer: This book draws on independent research commissioned by the National Institute for Health Research (NIHR). The views and opinions expressed by the interviewees in this publication are those of the interviewees and do not necessarily reflect those of the author, those of the NHS, the NIHR, MRC, CCF, NETSCC, the HS&DR programme or the Department of Health.

Policy Press works to counter discrimination on grounds of gender, race, disability, age and sexuality.

Cover design by Qube Design Associates, Bristol
Printed and bound in Great Britain by CMP, Poole
Policy Press uses environmentally responsible print partners

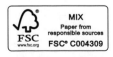

Contents

List of boxes, figures and tables

Boxes

Figures

Tables

Abbreviations

AAACM	all-age all-cause mortality
APMS	alternative provider medical services
CAA	comprehensive area assessment
CBA	cost-benefit analysis: a method of economic evaluation that compares costs and benefits in monetary terms
CCA	cost-consequence analysis: a method of economic evaluation that does not aggregate costs and consequences into a single metric and may include multiple and non-health-related outcomes across different sectors
CCG	clinical commissioning group
CEA	cost-effectiveness analysis: a method of economic evaluation that compares costs and outcomes and aims to achieve maximum gain, within available resources
CHC	community health council
CQC	Care Quality Commission
CQUIN	commissioning for quality and innovation
CSDH	Commission on Social Determinants of Health
CSR	comprehensive spending review
CUA	cost-utility analysis: a form of cost-effectiveness analysis which is used in the economic evaluation of health care interventions: effectiveness of interventions is assessed through a single index (quality of life). It is used by NICE to achieve consistent funding decisions
DALY	disability-adjusted life year
DPH	director of public health
FUR	freed-up resources
GMS	general medical services
GO	government office
HiAP	Health in All Policies
HWB	health and wellbeing board
JSNA	joint strategic needs assessment
LAA	local area agreement
LAT	local area team
LES	local enhanced service
LINk	local involvement network
LSP	local strategic partnership
NED	non-executive director
NICE	National Institute for Health and Care Excellence

NIHR	National Institute for Health Research
NIS	National Indicator Set
NPM	new public management
NSF	national service framework
OECD	Organisation for Economic Co-operation and Development
OSC	overview and scrutiny committee
P4P	pay for performance
PBC	practice-based commissioning
PBMA	programme budgeting and marginal analysis
PbR	payment by results
PCT	primary care trust
PEC	professional executive committee
PHICED	Public Health Interventions Cost-Effectiveness Database
PHS	preventative health spend
PMS	personal medical services: a locally agreed alternative to the general medical services (GMS) contract
PPI	patient and public involvement
PPIF	patient and public involvement forum
PSA	public service agreement
QALY	quality-adjusted life year
QIPP	Quality, Innovation, Productivity and Prevention
QOF	Quality and Outcomes Framework
ROI	return on investment
SHA	strategic health authority
SPOT	spend and outcome tool
VCS	voluntary and community sector
WCC	world class commissioning
WHO	World Health Organization

About the author

Linda Marks is senior research fellow in the Centre for Public Policy and Health, School of Medicine, Pharmacy and Health at Durham University. She has acted as an advisor for WHO Europe, as a non-executive director of a primary care trust in the NHS, and was formerly a health policy analyst at the King's Fund, London. A co-author of *The public health system in England* (Policy Press, 2010), she has published widely on public health policy and practice.

Acknowledgements

Governance, commissioning and public health forms part of the Evidence for Public Health Practice series and I would like to thank David Hunter and Stephen Peckham, the series editors, for their encouragement in writing this book. It arose from a research study, *Public health governance and primary care delivery: A triangulated study*, funded through the National Institute for Health Research (NIHR) Service Delivery and Organisation programme of research on public health (project no. 08/1716/208). Many people shaped the original research study, and the initial project team, which included David Hunter, Stephen Peckham, James Mason and Anna Coote, was gradually extended over the three years of the study. In particular, Sally Cave contributed greatly to the research and was responsible for carrying out much of the case study research across the country. Additional health economic support was contributed by Anne Mason and Helen Weatherly and I would like to acknowledge Anne Mason's analysis of theoretical approaches to incentives and Helen Weatherly's analysis of approaches to prioritisation in Chapters Five and Six. Andrew Wallace and Stephen Peckham carried out and analysed the national survey and Kate Melvin expertly carried out second-phase interviews. I would also like to thank her for her contribution to the chapter on public involvement in commissioning. Thanks to all of them for making the project possible – and also enjoyable.

The book draws on interview data gathered from a wide range of people as part of the study including NHS managers, non-executive directors, councillors, voluntary and community sector representatives, GPs and directors of public health, who generously gave up their time to be interviewed, to participate in surveys and in focus groups. I would like to express my appreciation to all of them, to the external advisory group for the study and to referees for their valuable feedback.

This book has been influenced by discussions with many people and by involvement in related public health research over the years. I would particularly like to thank Max Paddison, Andrew Gray, Tim Blackman, John Wilkinson, Richard Alderslade and Chris Brown – and would also like to acknowledge the formative influence of Peter Draper and colleagues at the former Unit for the Study of Health Policy, Guy's Hospital, London. Invaluable insights into commissioning were gained from experience as a non-executive director in the former Darlington Primary Care Trust and I would like to acknowledge the influence and support of Ken Greenfield and my former colleagues there.

The research was carried out at the Centre for Public Policy and Health, Durham University, and I would especially like to thank David Hunter, director of the Centre, for creating an environment where public health research has been consistently supported and encouraged.

Finally, views and opinions expressed in the book are those of the author (or of interviewees) and do not necessarily reflect those of the Department of Health, the NHS or the NIHR.

CHAPTER ONE

Introduction

Aspirations to 'move upstream' and invest for health are of long-standing – as are criticisms of national governments and local commissioners for failing to meet these aspirations. Investing for health involves action to prevent the causes of illness, shifting the focus from immediate, or proximate, causes of ill health (such as lifestyle factors) to the wider social, economic and environmental causes of ill health and health inequity, sometimes referred to as the 'the causes of the causes' (Rose, 1992). It also implies public health-informed policy, a longer-term perspective and a shift in investment priorities so that avoidable causes of morbidity and premature mortality can be addressed and health and wellbeing can be maximised. Given the nature of many public health challenges, success also depends on engagement of the public, building on community assets and strengths rather than focusing on deficits (Harrison et al., 2004; Foot and Hopkins, 2010), and encouraging wider policy and structural support for community activities that increase social capital and social cohesion (Putland et al., 2013).

These aspirations are reflected in national and international initiatives to reorient health and social care systems towards prevention and to encourage policy makers to address the social determinants of health and health equity. At an international level, efforts to prioritise prevention have gained prominence over the last forty years through a series of influential reports including the Canadian 'Lalonde' report (Lalonde, 1974) with its concept of the 'health field'; the Declaration of Alma Ata (WHO, 1978), which described health as a social goal; *Health for All by the year 2000* (WHO, 1981); and the *Ottawa charter for health promotion* (WHO, 1986). The latter reflected the breadth of public health action, spanning healthy public policy, community action and the reorientation of health care services towards the prevention of illness and the promotion of health. It also recognised the social determinants of health, emphasising that: 'the fundamental conditions and resources for health are peace, shelter, education, food, income, a stable eco-system, sustainable resources, social justice and equity'. This tradition continues through *Health 2020* (WHO 2012a), a European policy framework developed by the World Health Organization (WHO), and its associated *European action plan for strengthening public health capacities and services* (WHO, 2012b). *Health 2020* reaffirms the impact of social and economic factors on health and health equity but also emphasises that good health is fundamental for social and economic development: working across government is required to improve health and address health inequalities across the social gradient. These policy documents all make the case for greater priority being afforded to preventing ill health, reducing health inequalities and promoting population health.

The same themes have been reflected, to a greater or lesser extent, in an English policy context, with reports drawing together implications for the NHS and for the wider economy of failing to invest for health and emphasising the importance of addressing inequalities through action on the social determinants of health. Continuity of analysis (if not of policy implementation or of political commitment) can be traced from the materialist approach of the Black Report (1980), through the Acheson report on inequalities in health (Acheson, 1998) with its 39 recommendations across the whole of government, to the Labour government's broad-ranging *Tackling health inequalities: a programme for action* (Department of Health, 2003a) and the more recent strategic review of health inequalities in England, *Fair society, healthy lives* (Marmot Review, 2010), with its emphasis on reducing the social gradient in health across the life course.

Arguments based on social justice and fairness have been bolstered by economic arguments and the escalating costs associated with treatment and loss of productivity as a result of preventable morbidity. These themes were reflected in two influential reports commissioned by HM Treasury from Sir Derek Wanless (Wanless, 2002, 2004) where he argued the case for a better resourced and invigorated public health system, focusing attention on the benefits of a healthier population both in terms of reductions in the use of health and social care and in relation to the wider economy. This analysis was influential in increasing the funding allocation for the NHS by the Labour government (1997–2010) and policy documents produced during this period emphasised the importance of shifting the focus towards prevention (Secretary of State for Health, 2004, 2006; Department of Health, 2007a). However, the difficulties involved, even within the relatively narrow confines of the health sector and at a time of funding growth, were not underestimated. For example, the five year plan for the NHS (Secretary of State for Health, 2009) *NHS 2010–2015: From good to great. Preventative, people-centred, productive,* emphasised that nothing less than a 'paradigm shift' would be required. Some years earlier, the White Paper, *Our health, our care, our say* (Secretary of State for Health, 2006) had asserted that a shift was needed in the 'gravity of spending'.

Despite these repeated policy commitments at national and international levels, it has proved difficult to achieve this hoped-for 'paradigm shift' towards prevention or to narrow health inequalities, which are getting wider (Audit Commission, 2010; Marmot Review, 2010). This has been the case within the relatively narrow sphere of health care systems (Marks and Hunter, 2005), in the introduction of policies in other sectors which take account of health impact (Wismar et al., 2007) or in promoting social and economic policies which promote social justice and thereby reduce health inequalities. Many reasons have been suggested for this failure (see, for example, Mackenbach, 2010). Public health challenges, such as obesity (Butland et al., 2007) or health inequalities (Blackman et al., 2012) are inherently complex and involve simultaneous and concerted action across a range of sectors. The complexity of these challenges and their interconnectedness with commercial interests and the wider political and social environment militate against simple solutions: moreover, health inequalities cannot be considered separately from wider social and economic inequalities (Wilkinson and Pickett, 2010). A final reason is the scope and 'industrial' scale of interventions required to make a difference at a population level (Bentley, 2008). In practice, the health care sector has a high public and political profile, and its demands overshadow a longer-term public health agenda. Through associating public health systems with health systems, the scope of public health activity may be unintentionally narrowed (although it is possible that the relocation of public health responsibilities to local authorities in England from 2013 may go some way towards redressing this balance).

Questions are also raised over the adequacy of the evidence base for public health interventions, although, to some extent, this is a consequence of the complex nature of public health problems. The public health evidence base has been largely focused on lifestyle-related interventions, which partly accounts for the well-documented phenomenon of 'lifestyle drift' (Hunter et al., 2009), where an initial policy emphasis on economic and social determinants swiftly becomes translated into evidence-based, but narrower, interventions designed to change individual lifestyles. This is often associated with a focus on disadvantaged groups rather than on the social gradient in health (Milton et al., 2010). The methodological approach appropriate for evaluating health technologies is not best suited for evaluating complex community-based interventions and a sole emphasis on randomised controlled trials will work against the system-wide action which is often needed.

Despite these difficulties, the case has also been made that existing tools and levers are being inconsistently or inadequately applied (Bentley, 2008), and comparative reviews of public health performance and spending demonstrate that 'local strategies can work' (Audit Commission, 2010). There is, therefore, an important role for local commissioners.

In the context of the Labour government, a key route through which the 'shift in gravity' towards prevention was to be achieved locally was through NHS commissioning organisations. Primary care trusts (PCTs) held the major responsibility at the time for improving health and addressing health inequalities, which included working across local partnerships in recognition of the wider determinants of health. The publication of a *Commissioning framework for health and well-being* (Department of Health, 2007a) signalled the intention to help commissioners achieve a more strategic orientation towards promoting health and wellbeing, with a stronger focus on commissioning services and interventions across health and local government (para. 1.1) and 'shifting resources to where investment can have the greatest impact on current and future health and wellbeing needs' (para. 1.11). This was also intended to reduce future costs of ill health. These aspirations were subsequently reflected in the initiative for world class commissioning (WCC) (2007–10), which specified governance standards and health outcomes, and described the competencies needed by commissioners. It also incorporated a complex performance management framework for NHS commissioners (an aspect often perceived as overly burdensome).

However, shifting the focus of investment of local commissioning organisations towards prevention and addressing health inequalities also proved difficult (House of Commons Health Committee, 2009), despite the inexorable rise in non-communicable diseases, where many of the risk factors can be prevented and where early detection can reduce disability, morbidity and premature mortality. Weaknesses in the skills and capacity of local commissioners were cited as barriers, although this criticism may derive from an underestimate of the resources, incentives and political will required to carry out successful commissioning for public health in the face of competing demands. Short-term gains often prevail over the longer-term benefits of investment in public health for pragmatic and political reasons. Moreover, the public may not be 'fully engaged' with a local public health agenda, which has less immediacy than engaging with the quality and accessibility of local health and social care services. This can make cuts in local public health services a relatively easy option for commissioners.

But there are also signs of change. All health economies face increased costs due to the rising burden of non-communicable diseases and ageing populations: moral and ethical arguments for investment in prevention are increasingly bolstered by powerful economic arguments. There is a growing evidence base for cost–effective public health interventions (Owen et al., 2012), more emphasis on demonstrating 'return on investment' for preventive initiatives in local commissioning organisations (Matrix Insight, 2009a, 2011) and attempts to model the costs of preventable morbidity both for the NHS (Bernstein et al., 2010) and for the wider economy. For example, Butland et al. (2007) estimated costs of NHS treatment for obesity at £4.2 billion in 2007, with costs to the wider economy estimated at £15.8 billion. There is also encouragement for policy makers and local commissioners to develop joined-up strategies for addressing underlying determinants of health across the life course (Marmot Review, 2010) and a renewed emphasis on the social determinants of health and health equity. The relocation of public health into local authorities has the potential to put the 'public' back into public health (South et al., 2012) and encourage collective approaches to health improvement. In a context where health care costs are becoming unsustainable but where much ill health is preventable, local commissioning decisions reflect how much emphasis is being given, in practice, to prevention and to investing for health.

The public health governance study

This book draws on one of the public health research projects funded by the former National Institute for Health Research (NIHR) Service Delivery and Organisation (SDO) public health research programme. The research study *Public health governance and primary care delivery: A triangulated study* (Marks et al., 2011a) assessed the influence of governance structures and incentive arrangements on commissioning for health and wellbeing in the English NHS, as part of a wider programme of NIHR-funded research on 'incentives, performance and governance'. The study involved a range of research activities, including national and regional focus groups, a national survey of PCTs, and extensive fieldwork in 10 selected case study sites across England. Almost 100 interviews were carried out across PCTs, local authorities, general practices, the voluntary and community sector (VCS) and public involvement organisations (local involvement networks (LINks)), which had been set up in 2008. Each chapter draws on empirical research evidence gathered through the study and more details on the study design, including snapshots of the 10 case study sites, can be found in the Appendix.

The book builds on this research to illustrate how principles of governance (and the governance arrangements that are intended to flow from them) influence public health priorities through local decision making. Adopting a broad governance framework, it explores local commissioning practice during a period of concerted political commitment and policy action for improving health and addressing health inequalities, and which coincided with the implementation of WCC. Inevitably, its scope is somewhat limited by a focus on local organisations. The notion of 'commissioning for health and wellbeing', with its connotations of local assessment and service provision, sits uneasily with the influence of public policy on health, whether through housing, income distribution, welfare provision or education policy. The effectiveness of commissioners is inevitably affected by this wider political and economic context, and by the strength of government commitments to addressing social determinants of health and health equity through national policy. Improving health and wellbeing clearly reaches far beyond considerations of a commissioning cycle, decisions of any single commissioning organisation, the remit of public health services, or local partnerships. Despite this relatively narrow focus, decisions by commissioning organisations (however configured) remain an important influence and area for study, and illustrate questions of wider policy relevance. How do approaches to governance (separately and taken as a whole) influence population health? To what extent is a concern with public health reflected in governance arrangements, such as regulation, standards, incentives, targets and performance management regimes across different levels of decision making? How are notions of collective responsibility or a stewardship role reflected in local organisations and partnerships?

At a local level, the answers to these questions lie in how commissioning for health and wellbeing is understood and operationalised, the priority attached to a preventive agenda and the matrix of regulations, protocols, targets and incentives within which commissioners make decisions. Through exploring how governance principles and arrangements shape how commissioning for health and wellbeing is understood and prioritised, the study develops 'public health governance' as a critical concept.

Changing commissioning contexts for public health

There have been major changes in the context and accountability arrangements for commissioning since the study was completed in 2010. At the time of the study (2007–10), 152 PCTs across England controlled about 80% of the NHS budget and were responsible for commissioning primary, secondary and community health services, including preventive health services. Directors of public health (DsPH) were accountable to PCTs (although many were joint appointments across PCTs and local authorities). Partnership working across a local authority area was arranged through non-statutory, multi-agency local strategic partnerships (LSPs), bringing together key partners from the public, private and voluntary sectors. From 2004, the involvement of general practice in NHS commissioning had been encouraged through 'practice-based commissioning' (PBC), where general practices were incentivised to work with PCTs to develop commissioning strategies (although with variable success).

Since 2010, there have been major changes in the organisation and commissioning of public health services in England as part of a far-reaching, contested and largely unanticipated reorganisation of the NHS (Timmins, 2012) culminating, after a two-year process, in the Health and Social Care Act 2012. The coalition government's White Paper, *Equity and excellence: Liberating the NHS* (Secretary of State for Health, 2010a), introduced new, statutory general practice consortia (later renamed clinical commissioning groups [CCGs]) which replaced PCTs as the main commissioning organisations for the NHS. Accountable to a new national body, NHS England, they are responsible for 65% of the NHS budget, commissioning services for planned hospital care, rehabilitative care, urgent and emergency care, most community health services, maternity services, mental health and learning disability services. Some NHS services, including primary care services, dental and ophthalmic services, national public health services such as immunisation and vaccination, and specialised services are commissioned by NHS England. Public health responsibilities of PCTs were shifted from the NHS to democratically elected local authorities, supported by a new and independent executive agency of the Department of Health, Public Health England. Reflecting the situation prior to the 1974 reorganisation of the NHS, local authorities reclaimed the major responsibility for public health commissioning and DsPH and their teams were duly transferred to local authorities from April 2013, when the reforms were implemented. The public health White Paper, *Healthy lives, healthy people* (Secretary of State for Health,

2010b), published four months after *Equity and excellence*, clarified public health functions and responsibilities of unitary and upper-tier local authorities, the support to be provided by Public Health England, and the role of new health and wellbeing boards (HWBs). The latter were statutory committees of the local authority with core membership to include at least one local authority councillor, the director of adult social services, the director of children's services, a representative of local Healthwatch, the DPH and a member of each CCG, with other members co-opted according to local discretion.

The relocation of responsibility for public health from the NHS to local authorities was widely welcomed as a move towards a social model of health (House of Commons Communities and Local Government [CLG] Committee, 2013) with decisions made in a context of local democratic accountability. The reforms reaffirmed the importance of localism and served to emphasise the public health role of local authorities through their influence on broader determinants of health, such as housing and the environment. They resulted in the transfer from the NHS of a ring-fenced public health grant for commissioning a wide range of public health preventive activities including tobacco control, health checks, alcohol and drug misuse, physical activity, mental health, sexual health and environmental risk (Department of Health, 2011a, 2012d): it was anticipated that these changes in commissioning responsibilities would encourage innovative approaches to improving health and addressing health inequalities. From April 2015, responsibilities for the Healthy Child Programme (health visiting services and the family nurse partnership programme) would also transfer, giving local authorities more influence across the life course. Effectiveness of the reforms would depend not only on how the ring-fenced budget was deployed, but also on the extent to which new public health responsibilities were reflected across local authority directorates. The House of Commons CLG Committee (2013: para. 88) noted that:

> Local authorities, if they are to grasp fully the opportunity afforded to them by the return of public health, will need to look beyond those services traditionally considered to be 'public health', such as health protection, health promotion and disease prevention, and tackle the causes of the causes of poor health, working with local partners and using all the powers, personnel and services at their disposal.

Despite these major changes in organisation and accountability, there were similarities with arrangements prior to 2013. CCGs (211 at the time of writing) built on the organisations developed through PBC and gradually adopted many of the responsibilities of the PCTs they replaced; joint strategic needs assessments (JSNAs), established in 2008 to assess health and wellbeing needs and health inequalities in local populations, were retained but became the responsibility of the new HWBs, along with new joint health and wellbeing strategies. HWBs replaced a mixed array of health and wellbeing partnerships, were placed on a statutory footing and included CCGs as core members.

While WCC was discontinued by the coalition government in 2010, their public health White Paper, *Healthy lives, healthy people* (Secretary of State for Health, 2010b), continued to emphasise the importance of prevention and addressing health inequalities. The four domains of a new public health outcomes framework (Department of Health, 2012a) provided indicators against which local authorities could assess their performance, but no specific targets were set and the emphasis shifted from the detailed performance management arrangements of the previous government towards local self-assessment. However, a reorientation towards prevention, partnership working and 'investing to save' continue to be emphasised in public health strategies.

Whatever the context and accountability arrangements for commissioning, policy makers and public health commissioners face a number of generic questions. How are the needs of the local population to be assessed? How far is a concern with health and health inequalities reflected throughout the commissioning process? To what extent is the public involved in commissioning? How are priorities identified in practice and then reflected in commissioning decisions? What is the influence of policy mandates, the pattern of incentives across a system and governance arrangements, including those for audit and scrutiny? These questions are addressed in the course of the book.

Governance, commissioning and public health: definitions

Each of these key concepts – governance, commissioning and public health – is subject to multiple interpretations, and parameters vary according to the contexts in which they are used. The following section, therefore, briefly outlines these concepts before exploring their mutual relevance. Subsequent chapters explore these themes in more detail, drawing on research evidence gathered through the study.

Governance and 'good governance'

As further described in Chapter Two, governance is open to many different interpretations. While governance arrangements provide a key route for achieving goals and objectives, whether for national government or for local organisations, the term 'governance' and its parameters are notoriously elusive (Rhodes, 1996; Davies et al., 2005). Principles of governance, such as accountability or equity, may be uncontentious, but the extent to which these principles are reflected in governance arrangements (such as performance management), the effectiveness of such arrangements and the impact of modes of governance, such as markets or networks, are all open to debate. One of the arguments put forward in this book is that each of the dimensions of governance is relevant for understanding local commissioning practice in relation to health and wellbeing, and that these dimensions can usefully be considered separately, although they operate as a whole. For example, 'good governance' has been used to refer to governance based on underlying principles, including accountability, participation and social justice (Weiss, 2000). Governance arrangements provide a means through which such underlying principles may be operationalised via a wide range of 'steering instruments', including policies, standards and targets, and through mechanisms for audit, scrutiny and regulation. However, governance arrangements may not reflect underlying principles, there may be a lack of alignment across national, regional and local levels of governance, or specific instruments of governance may exert perverse or unintended consequences and therefore not fulfil their intended purpose.

The importance of understanding how different approaches to governance can affect population health and health equity, and the key importance of social justice as a governance principle have become increasingly recognised. Both are reflected in *Health 2020*, WHO Europe's health policy framework (WHO, 2012a), which emphasises the importance of collaboration and co-governance for promoting public health in the 21st century (building on underpinning documents on 'governance for health' [Kickbusch and Gleicher, 2012] and on the social determinants of health and health equity across the European Region [Marmot, 2013]). *Health 2020* is a response to widening health inequalities within countries and across Europe, the growing impact of non-communicable diseases, and the social and economic causes of health and health inequity, as described in the earlier influential report of the WHO Global Commission on Social Determinants of Health (CSDH), *Closing the gap in a generation* (WHO, 2008). *Health 2020* emphasises addressing health inequity, that is, 'differences which are not only unnecessary and avoidable but in addition are considered unfair and unjust' (Whitehead, 1992), and the unequal distribution of the social determinants of health, such as housing, education and income. This directly relates to governance principles of social justice, the importance attached to health as a human right and the extent to which these principles are reflected in policy making across government.

Population health is, therefore, inextricably linked with the broad spectrum of public policy which influences these determinants and inequalities in health arise from their unequal distribution across the population. An emphasis on equity, combined with a recognition of the influence of public policy on health and the importance of 'whole of government' approaches, points to the key influence of governance – in particular, the principles underlying governance – on health. It raises questions over how these principles are reflected in instruments of governance, such as law and policy, and whether these instruments are effectively implemented.

Governance is often associated with hierarchies, networks and markets, although partnership and participatory approaches to governance are of particular relevance for addressing public health challenges, which often involve working across networks of different stakeholders (at national and local levels) and need to build on effective citizen engagement. As discussed in the third book in this series (Hunter and Perkins, 2014) and in Chapter Two, multisectoral working and partnerships also create governance challenges, reflecting the difficulties of working across organisations with different budgets, priorities and accountabilities. *Health 2020* reiterates the importance of 'whole of government', and multisectoral approaches to improving health, also emphasising that this needs to be accompanied by a 'whole of society' approach, encompassing citizen engagement and participation.

Modes of governance are associated with different 'steering instruments', including targets, audit arrangements and incentives, and the balance adopted across regulatory and other approaches is influenced by the political context. However, certain steering instruments may not be appropriate when applied to complex systems and can lead to unforeseen consequences. As discussed in Chapter Four, centrally driven targets for reducing health inequalities, in place from 2002 to 2010, were not always prioritised in practice, and the need to demonstrate 'quick wins' led to an emphasis on clinical preventive interventions, rather than on the longer-term action required to address social determinants of health (Blackman et al., 2012). Moreover, the relationship between 'steering instruments' and modes of governance is complex and it has been pointed out (Saltman, 2002) that decentralisation and the adoption of market-style incentives serves to increase the regulatory role of government in health care systems, rather than the reverse.

Commissioning for health and wellbeing

Commissioning is also subject to interpretation, as is the popular phrase 'commissioning for health and wellbeing', and these are discussed in turn. 'Commissioning' in the health sector has been understood in different ways since the term gained currency during the 1990s and, perhaps not surprisingly, the ramifications of the term remain largely obscure to the general public (House of Commons Health Committee, 2010: para. 1). Although the aim of planning services in relation to need has been in existence as long as the NHS, 'commissioning' is largely associated with public sector reforms dating from the 1990s, which promoted the separation of purchasing from the provision of services (otherwise known as the 'purchaser/provider split'), described in detail elsewhere (see, for example, House of Commons Health Committee 2010, 2011; Glasby, 2012). In England, commissioning activities and arrangements in the NHS reflect political views over the role of markets, choice and competitive tendering as a source of quality. They are, therefore, particularly prone to being reorganised in the context of political change and repeated reorganisations can, in themselves, make it difficult to demonstrate progress. Commissioning arrangements reflect different positions over the role of regulation, the role of a market-based system in health care and the degree of private sector involvement in the delivery of NHS-funded services. They also reflect different views over the balance to be achieved across clinical and managerial influence, the appropriate size and structure of commissioning organisations, and how accountability is to be achieved. In this sense, commissioning arrangements both reflect and embody different modes of governance which, in turn, have an impact on how commissioning for health and wellbeing is understood and implemented locally. In the devolved administrations of Scotland and Wales, for example, England's quasi-market approach has been rejected and the purchaser/provider split dismantled. In Wales, seven local health boards are responsible for both planning and providing hospital, primary and community care, in line with policies set by the Welsh government (Longley et al., 2012), while in Scotland, planning and provision of services is provided through 14 integrated NHS boards, with an emphasis on partnership and integration. Community health partnerships (committees of NHS boards) are responsible for primary and community care (Steel and Cylus, 2012).

In England, *The NHS plan* (Secretary of State for Health, 2000) had identified a lack of national standards, over-centralisation and a 'lack of clear incentives and levers to improve performance' (p. 10). Over the decade that followed, commissioning practice was shaped by a wide range of levers, including national standards, contractual flexibilities, policies for patient choice, PBC, the introduction of payment by results (where money was intended to 'follow the patient') and the initiative for WCC, intended to focus on health outcomes. These were all supported by a complex system of regulation, targets and incentives which were sometimes interrelated and mutually reinforcing, but often contradictory and ill aligned. Despite the sentiments expressed in the *NHS plan*, these new arrangements were themselves often criticised as over-centralised.

The substantial demands and transactional costs involved in contracting for health care services have tended to preserve and foster a narrow definition of commissioning as largely comprising purchasing and contract specification. In contrast to this, WCC was intended to promote the commissioning cycle as a whole, commissioning for improved health outcomes, service quality and value for money across a total budget, as opposed to concentrating on one part of that cycle, the transactional phase. WCC set out a continuous cycle of needs assessment, gap analysis, service specification, and the purchasing of services which were then monitored and evaluated, before the cycle was repeated. There were 11 commissioning competencies: commissioners were required to work with community partners, engage with the public and patients, and, as part of 'prioritising investment', to develop transparent investment decision-making processes. They were also required to identify and tackle 'inequalities of health status, access and resource allocation' (Department of Health, 2007b: 3). In this model, needs assessment was intended as the cornerstone of a commissioning strategy, and, although the reality may often have differed due to other pressures, the commissioning cycle provided an opportunity to address heath inequalities, gaps in services and also recognise the social determinants of health at a local level. This is further discussed in Chapter Three, which considers the commissioning cycle and, in particular, the JSNA, in more detail.

The emphasis in the NHS has largely remained on arrangements for commissioning health care services and on attempts to redress the balance between relatively weak commissioners on the one hand and more powerful provider organisations (NHS Trusts, in England) on the other. Commissioning in social care, joint commissioning across health and social services or commissioning related to public health and preventive services have been relatively neglected (Glasby and Dickinson, 2014; Hunter and Perkins, 2014). The initiative for 'commissioning for health and wellbeing' through WCC could, therefore, be seen as encouraging a change in emphasis. However, the phrase is also something of a 'catch-all', with an interpretation to suit every purpose. Arguably, the entire range of activities carried out by health and social care commissioning organisations (and many outside the health sector) could be included under the broad rubric of 'commissioning for health and wellbeing', in the sense of promoting health, recovery, rehabilitation or independence. The phrase can also refer to providing preventive and integrated care organised around individual needs, or reducing the need for hospital admission. It may equally be interpreted as preventing ill health through a range of specific preventive services, such as smoking cessation or the promotion of physical activity. These may be focused on individual lifestyle change or on the creation of an environment which promotes healthier choices. Given the phrase allows for multiple interpretations and emphases, its use can lead to fudging of priorities and even to the neglect of a preventive agenda.

Although often used synonymously with health, 'wellbeing' is distinct from health status, and subject to cultural and social construction. Subjective wellbeing has been adopted as a government goal and 10 'general wellbeing' indicators are being developed by the Office for National Statistics for use in attitudinal surveys. Practical and resource guides have also been produced (Michaelson et al., 2012). This reflects similar initiatives in Europe, and elsewhere, to redefine what is meant by societal wellbeing, including factors such as social cohesion, in attempts to move the emphasis away from narrow economic indicators related to economic growth. In the UK, health, employment status and relationship status are among factors most highly associated with wellbeing (Office for National Statistics, 2013). While local commissioners are clearly limited in their capacity to influence the range of national influences on wellbeing, both CCGs and local authorities can play a key role in promoting local health and community wellbeing.

Public health definitions

As discussed in detail in the first book in the series, *The public health system in England* (Hunter et al., 2010), 'definitions of public health abound, varying between times and contexts' (p. 18). Public health can refer to the health of populations, the public health function (incorporating health protection, health promotion and heath service improvement), the public health profession or a public health system. The parameters of a public health system are also open to debate depending on the nature of the public health issue under consideration, the workforce and organisations involved in addressing it, and the extent of cross-sectoral action required. For example, a concern with wider social and economic factors may be limited to addressing the health impact of specific social factors, such as housing, or be broad in scope, including impacts on population health of climate change, cultural change or globalisation (McMichael et al., 2006; Hanlon and Carlisle, 2008; Hanlon et al., 2011; Frenk and Moon, 2013). The complex causation of public health threats needs to be reflected in the ways that health systems and public health systems are conceptualised (Hunter et al., 2010; Marks et al., 2011b) and in the range of organisational responses that would be required. Public health problems share the same ambiguity of definition. Verweij and Dawson (2007) point out, for example, that characterising an issue as a public health problem can mean increasing incidence (an epidemiological issue); influenced by socioeconomic or other conditions (a causative issue); or requiring an urgent response, where action is in the public interest (a normative issue). Gaps between the social and economic conditions required for a healthy population and the activities of public health systems (however defined) or public health practitioners mean that debates over the definitions and scope of public health activity are inherently value based and politically contingent.

The definition of public health generally includes a future orientation and the notion of collective action in the public interest. Although many definitions have been put forward (see review in Marks et al., 2011b), the definition adopted by Sir Donald Acheson in 1988 has been widely accepted as reflecting the essence of public health but without narrowing its scope. His definition (following that of Winslow [1920]) described public health as follows: 'Public health is the science and art of preventing disease, prolonging life and promoting health through the organised efforts of society' (Acheson, 1988).

The theme of collective action, reflected in Acheson's definition of public health as involving 'the organised efforts of society', recognises the role of policy across sectors and implies action on the social determinants of health and of health equity. 'Organised efforts of society' also points to the link between public health and governance arrangements.

The Acheson definition refers to both the science and the 'art' of public health. Notwithstanding a growing evidence base for cost-effective public health interventions (Owen et al., 2012), the 'art' of public health recognises the complexity of public health challenges, influenced by political, cultural and commercial factors and, in light of this, the inevitable limitations of an evidence base which is concerned with specific public health interventions. Understanding the social determinants of health and health equity involves analysing corporate interests on patterns of consumption, political commitments to social justice and the distributional aspects of policies related to social determinants of health, such as housing, income and education. The Foresight report on obesity, for example, demonstrated the social, political, environmental and cultural action that would be required to address obesity, a multidimensional and complex public health problem with many interconnected causes (Butland et al., 2007). It meant adopting a system-wide approach, addressing multiple levels of influence simultaneously with a wide range of policy sectors and stakeholders. The uncertainty associated with many public health challenges is reflected in the notion of the 'precautionary principle' and the necessity of taking action, given the potential consequences of inaction, even in the absence of conclusive evidence (Martuzzi and Tickner, 2004).

While the scope and function of the public health profession, the public health function and a public health system have been variously defined over time, analysis of the governance implications that follow from the goals of maximising population health, developing local public health systems or addressing health inequalities, remains relatively neglected.

Public health and governance: shared values

Preventing avoidable ill health and promoting wellbeing are core public health values and clearly linked with wider values of social justice and human rights (Saracci, 2007; Gostin, 2008). The action required reaches far beyond public health systems, however broadly defined, to encompass public policy at national and international levels. The obligation to support the 'right to health', as part of an international commitment to human rights, is emphasised as a rationale and justification for promoting population health: the interconnectedness of health and of human rights has become increasingly prominent.

Entitlement to health as a human right is reflected in the Universal Declaration of Human Rights (adopted by the United Nations General

Assembly in 1948), in the 1946 Constitution of WHO, which states that the 'enjoyment of the highest attainable standard of health is one of the fundamental rights of every human being' and is further developed in the UN International Covenant on Economic, Social and Cultural Rights (UN General Assembly, 1966: Article 12). This commitment is also reflected in *Health 2020*. Agreements are associated with government obligations to move towards a 'progressive realisation' of the right to health (Yamin, 2008). What this means, in practice, is that policy across government should be informed by this governance principle. This was emphasised in a revised definition of the 'health in all policies' approach (originally described by Ståhl et al., 2006), as agreed at the Global Conference on Health Promotion in May 2013. This new definition reiterates connections between health and health equity, public policy and the right to health.

> Health in All Policies [HiAP] is an approach to public policies across sectors that systematically takes into account the health implications of decisions, seeks synergies, and avoids harmful health impacts in order to improve population health and health equity. A Health in All Policies approach is founded on health-related rights and obligations. It improves accountability of policy makers for health impacts at all levels of policy making. It includes an emphasis on the consequences of public policies on health systems, determinants of health, and wellbeing. (The Helsinki Statement on Health in all Policies, 2013)[1]

As the above quotation makes clear, the principles of good governance and the aims of achieving the highest attainable level of health and of addressing health inequity are crucially linked. One of the critical identifiers of whether a country exhibits 'good governance' is, therefore, the state of the health of its population: a 'stewardship' role in relation to population health has been presented as a key responsibility of government (Omaswa and Boufford, 2010). This has been characterised as 'the careful and responsible management of the wellbeing of the population ... the very essence of good government. The health of people is always a national priority: government responsibility for it is continuous and permanent' (WHO, 2000: viii).

Closely associated with concepts of governance, stewardship is also open to different interpretations, including being entrusted with responsibilities (as in financial stewardship); protection of the public interest by government; or as a form of corporate governance. The concept of 'system stewardship' has been developed to reflect problems of governance in complex systems and has been defined as 'policy makers overseeing the ways in which the policy is being adapted, and attempting to steer the system towards certain outcomes' (Hallsworth, 2011: 8). Perhaps reflecting the complexity of the current arrangements, the Department of Health describes its role as that of 'system steward', as 'the only body with oversight over the whole health and care system' (Department of Health, 2013c: 25).

National and local health-related organisations often reflect a stewardship role in relation to population health in their mission statements, goals and objectives, although whether health improvement and health equity are prioritised through governance arrangements and commissioning practice is another matter. Unless there is commitment to these principles at national government level, they are unlikely to be prioritised at a local level. What a stewardship role involves in practice also raises ethical and political debates over the balance to be achieved between collective approaches to public health, such as regulation and public health law, and individual responsibility and choice. These issues are revisited in the concluding chapter.

Plan of the book

Public health governance has been defined as 'the means by which society collectively seeks to assure the conditions under which the population can live with the highest possible level of health and wellbeing' (Institute of Medicine, 2002, quoted in Bennett et al., 2009). It has often been taken to refer to direct and indirect regulation by governments in the interests of population health. Drawing on different dimensions of governance, the notion of 'public health governance' is developed as a critical concept for assessing the extent to which a focus on health and wellbeing is reflected in underlying values informing decision making, priorities for investment, performance management arrangements, and in the use of incentives and contracts. Dimensions of governance are discussed in Chapter Two, with a particular emphasis on accountability arrangements, partnerships and the stewardship role.

Chapter Three looks in more detail at the commissioning cycle and discusses what is involved in a developing a public health-led approach to commissioning. This includes approaches to health needs assessment through the JSNA and JHWS and the engagement of general practice.

Chapters Four and Five are related, reviewing the influence of governance arrangements and incentives on commissioning for health and wellbeing. Incentives are often contingent on governance structures (such as incentives and reward schemes for reaching targets, for example) and modes of governance have implications for the kinds of incentives which are promoted. It has been argued, for example, that the particular mix of regulatory requirements and incentives (in the sense of inducements) is an indicator of the degree of state or market orientation (Saltman, 2002). Chapter Four reviews governance arrangements, including performance management regimes, their influence on decision making and their alignment across different agencies. The coalition government introduced major changes in this area and implications of these changes are discussed. Chapter Five explores links between governance approaches and the use of incentives, drawing on economic perspectives on incentives. It provides an account of incentives and contractual flexibilities used by commissioners to promote preventive services, in particular, local enhanced services (part of the new general medical services [GMS] contract introduced in 2004). Benefits and drawbacks of using incentives for public health services are discussed, drawing on interviews carried out as part of the study.

Chapter Six considers priority setting and issues which arise in attempting to shift the 'gravity of spend' in health-related organisations towards prevention. Whether policy is translated into practice depends on local decision-making and prioritisation processes. Different forms of 'evidence' come into play, along with different decision support methods and systems for reaching judgements. These include policy evaluation, the public health evidence base, different approaches to economic evaluation, option appraisal and impact assessments (environmental, social, health and health inequality). Drawing on local experience, approaches to prioritising investment and the applicability of current prioritisation methods and tools for longer-term public health investment are reviewed.

Improvements in population health are unlikely to be achieved without the involvement of the public. Participation by the public and accountability to the public are two key underlying principles of governance and, as such, need to be reflected in commissioning arrangements. However, public involvement in commissioning preventive services, as opposed to health and social care services, proved difficult for PCTs to achieve at the time of the study. Chapter Seven explores public involvement in commissioning for health and wellbeing, including the impact of changes arising from the creation of Healthwatch England and local Healthwatch, following implementation of the Health and Social Care Act 2012.

The conclusions draw themes together under the broad umbrella of 'public health governance' and future directions for commissioning are discussed.

Note

[1] See: www.who.int/healthpromotion/conferences/8gchp/statement_2013/en/

CHAPTER TWO

Dimensions of governance

This chapter considers the concept of governance and its relevance for population health and commissioning practice. It argues that governance for population health needs to be considered in relation to each of the dimensions of governance, which are briefly described. It then illustrates these dimensions through a discussion of stewardship of the health of the population, accountability arrangements, a partnership mode of governance and approaches to corporate governance, drawing on study data from interviews and focus groups. The concept of 'public health governance' is discussed, and returned to in the concluding chapter.

Governance: a multidimensional concept

Governance is a multidimensional and somewhat slippery concept and, as many commentators have pointed out (Rhodes, 1996; Weiss, 2000; Davies et al., 2005), it is subject to diverse interpretations. In general, it refers to the 'totality of ways in which a society organises and collectively manages its affairs' (Frenk and Moon, 2013: 937, drawing on discussion in United Nations Development Programme, 1997). It incorporates notions of the proper functioning of institutions, the exercise of legitimate authority and the arrangements organisations (of any kind) make for their functioning: governance arrangements are organised routes for achieving objectives, whatever the level or form of organisation involved. An underpinning document for *Health 2020* (WHO, 2012a) refers to governance as 'how governments and other social organisations interact, how they relate to citizens and how decisions are taken in a complex world' (Kickbusch and Gleicher, 2012: 1, quoting Graham et al., 2003). Such decisions may be operationalised through market mechanisms, networks or hierarchies, sometimes referred to as 'modes' of governance although, in practice, these are ideal types: modes may coexist; the relative emphasis on each may fluctuate over time; and, as in the NHS, they exist in hybrid forms. Moreover, other forms of governance, such as multilevel governance, have become increasingly important given the combination of international with national and regional levels of authority. Governance may be associated with a set of principles ('good governance'), codes of conduct in public life, the exercise of legitimate authority through law and regulation, standards and targets, and processes for ensuring accountability and managing risk within organisations. It may also apply to the systematic application of procedures to a particular topic (as in 'clinical governance' or 'digital governance'). At an organisational level, corporate governance has been a common focus of governance-related research, often triggered by serious 'governance deficits' which have come to light in corporations, such as those which led to the collapse of the Enron corporation in 2001, and in the NHS, by the failures of clinical care in Mid-Staffordshire NHS Trust between 2005 and 2009 (Francis Inquiry, 2010, 2013), with estimates of almost five hundred excess deaths. The latter provided an example of how certain aspects of governance, in this case meeting financial targets, dominated at the expense of core values of the organisation, to provide good quality care.

There have been numerous attempts to categorise and delineate different dimensions of governance, including ways in which 'governance' can be distinguished from 'government'; the genesis of the notion of 'good governance' in international development (Weiss, 2000); the impact of modes of governance on outcomes; and the combination of governance arrangements most likely to improve performance. Governance studies span underlying values, instruments of governance and a gamut of decision-making arrangements at different levels of organisation, drawing on organisational theory, policy and public administration studies, human rights research and political science. A single definition of governance is, therefore, elusive.

A review of governance issues of relevance to NHS boards (NHS National Leadership Council, 2010: 40) argued that 'a sound understanding of governance derives from assimilating and blending this range of perspectives', the perspectives in this case comprising five 'models' of governance including: an agency model, which includes performance management regimes, incentives and sanctions; a stakeholder model, which involves engaging and balancing a multiplicity of stakeholder views; a stewardship model which engages with civic society through developing a framework of shared values; policy governance which distinguishes between the public and those who deliver services on its behalf within a policy framework; and 'generative governance', which involves active dialogue across board, staff and users.

Table 2.1 summarises different dimensions of governance and the rest of the chapter considers their relevance for commissioning and decision making for population health.

Table 2.1: Dimensions of governance

Dimensions of Governance	Examples				
Principles/ values	Social justice Human rights Stewardship - health - economy - environment	Conduct - seven principles of conduct in public life (Nolan principles)	Good governance in public services - promoting values and a focus on purpose and outcomes	Accountability Transparency	Participation
Governance arrangements/ processes	Allocation of authority - roles and responsibilities - law and regulation - rights	Standards, targets and performance management regimes	Accountability arrangements - professional /public/ democratic - vertical/ horizontal	Processes for ensuring transparency, effectiveness and managing risk	Audit and inspection
Modes of governance	Hierarchies (agency model)	Networks (stakeholder model) / co-governance /partnership governance	Markets (contractual)	Hybrid forms	Participatory governance
Levels of governance	Global to local	System	Organisational (corporate governance)	Multilevel-dispersed authority and decision making	Community/ neighbourhood governance
Topic-based/ functions (examples)	Clinical governance	Information governance	Digital governance	Carbon governance	Public health governance

Source: Adapted from Marks et al. (2011c); reprinted with permission from the *Journal of Health Services Research and Policy* 16 (Suppl. 1).

While illustrating the complexity of governance, Table 2.1 also provides a framework for 'interrogating' dimensions of governance in relation to their impact on population health and health equity. For example, questions could include the following:

- How is stewardship of the health of the population defined and then operationalised through governance arrangements?
- Do decision-making processes reflect a commitment to an underlying governance principle of promoting population health and health equity?

- Is there clarity over what is to be achieved at each level of governance (national, regional, local) and is there effective coordination and integration across these different levels?
- Do governance arrangements for commissioning organisations, such as scrutiny and audit, adequately reflect duties and priorities in relation to health improvement and addressing health inequalities?
- To what extent is there alignment across performance management arrangements, corporate risk management, financial strategies and commissioning priorities in relation to population health?
- Are governance arrangements in place for ensuring accountability to the public in relation to commissioning for health and wellbeing and for prevention of ill health?
- How is the public involved in shaping decisions related to population health?

While these topics are considered in more detail in the following chapters, this chapter summarises key debates in relation to the dimensions of governance suggested in Table 2.1 and discusses examples.

Underlying principles of governance

> Health is considered a human right, an essential component of wellbeing, a global public good and an issue of social justice and equity. (Kickbusch and Gleicher, 2012: viii)

Normative judgements inherent in a notion of 'good governance' have been contested as not fundamental to the study of governance, originally value neutral and derived from accounting procedures. However, 'good governance' is increasingly used as a short-hand term for governance which reflects widely accepted social values and which usually involves a combination of such values. These include the human right to health, social justice, accountability, participation and transparency (although distinctions between certain values, such as accountability and transparency are themselves blurred and the subject of debate [Hood, 2010]). This has led to debate over what is meant by 'good governance' in different contexts and the values that underpin and shape governance arrangements. Principles of good governance have been considered in relation to international decision making, public bodies, including the English NHS, and standards of conduct in public life. The Independent Commission on Good Governance in Public Services (2004) noted that 'good governance leads to good management, good performance, good stewardship of public money, good public engagement and, ultimately, good outcomes' (p. v). Building on principles for the conduct of individuals in public life ('Nolan principles') (Committee on Standards in Public Life, 1995) it outlined six core principles of good governance:

- focusing on the organisation's purpose and on outcomes for citizens and service users;
- performing effectively in clearly defined functions and roles;
- promoting values for the whole organisation and demonstrating the values of good governance through behaviour;
- taking informed, transparent decisions and managing risk;
- developing the capacity and capability of the governing body to be effective;
- engaging stakeholders and making accountability real.

Various international organisations, including the Organisation for Economic Co-operation and Development (OECD) (Oman and Arndt, 2010) and the United Nations Development Programme (1997) have attempted to classify and measure 'good governance'. For example, the Worldwide Governance Indicators Project,[1] developed through the World Bank, includes six broad dimensions of governance, namely: voice and accountability; political stability and absence of violence; government effectiveness; regulatory quality; rule of law; and control of corruption. This allows for an assessment of governance arrangements across countries.

Governance studies also highlight challenges involved in 'good global governance', where coordinated global action is required to address current and emerging problems. Global public health challenges include climate change, the consequences on health and other sectors of the globalisation of markets, finance and labour, and what Frenk and Moon (2013) have described as an 'unfinished agenda' of infection, malnutrition and maternal conditions, and the rise of non-communicable diseases. They all involve multilevel action and multi-agency working, where regional, national, supranational and transnational levels of decision making may need to come into play, as well as the participation of local communities. In recognition of this, the Commission on Social Determinants of Health (CSDH) argues that 'in a globalised world, the need for governance dedicated to equity applies equally from the community level to global institutions' (WHO, 2008: 44). The Lancet-University of Oslo Commission on Global Governance for Health re-emphasised that 'grave health inequity is morally unacceptable' (Ottersen et al., 2014: 661) and argued that improved global governance was urgently required to address the power disparities associated with transnational activities which comprised what the Commission described as 'the global political determinants of health'. Health and health equity are, therefore, considered to lie at the heart of governance, with health equity considered as a marker of government performance and social justice as a hallmark of good governance. This, in turn, implies a commitment to address social and economic influences on health equity in national strategies and policies and across partnerships. Policy coherence across different departments of government (reflected in aligned governance arrangements) is of key importance, as is a process for identifying the health (and health equity) impact of policies – and then acting on the results (Kemm and Parry, 2004). For example, 'Health in All Policies' (HiAP) aims to ensure that a health dimension is integrated into activities of all European Commission services, through methods such as health impact assessment. This brings together economic, social and environmental impacts in a single mechanism (Ståhl et al., 2006). Stewardship in this context may involve trade-offs across different sectors and reflects political choices and priorities.

In its opening statement, CSDH reiterates the impact of social and economic policies on life chances and squarely locates these issues within an agenda for social justice:

> The development of a society, rich or poor, can be judged by the quality of its population's health, how fairly health is distributed across the social spectrum, and the degree of protection provided from disadvantage as a result of ill health. (WHO, 2008)

This approach was applied to England in *Fair society, healthy lives* (Marmot Review, 2010), which outlined priority objectives and policy recommendations across six key policy areas in order to address entrenched health inequalities. Instigated under the Labour government, the findings of the Marmot Review were subsequently accepted by the 2010 coalition government.

As noted in the introduction, the notion of 'good governance' is closely associated with the stewardship role of the state with regard to the health of the population. At national level, the ways in which the stewardship role of government is discharged influence the extent to which a concern with the health of populations permeates policy development, health impact assessment, priority setting and decision making. It may be reflected in the balance between 'upstream' and 'downstream' interventions; the extent to which prevention of ill health and the reduction of inequalities are resourced and prioritised; and levels of citizen engagement and social inclusion. Stewardship therefore raises questions over the primacy of health and health improvement in decisions taken in other policy sectors which may have a bearing on health. A stewardship role is not limited to national government but is also reflected at a local organisational level and the following section discusses how this role was understood in the study.

A stewardship role: views from the study

In the study, commitment to public health values was indicated by the relative emphasis accorded to specific targets, partnership working, the use of incentives for preventive services and the extent to which investment in health and wellbeing was prioritised.

Local authorities already had a duty to promote social, economic and environmental wellbeing through their community strategies, as set out in the Local Government Act 2000, while the first of the three main functions of primary care trusts (PCTs) at the time of the study was to engage with the local population to improve health and wellbeing (Department of Health, 2006a). This had three elements:

• Improving the health status of its population, and reducing health inequalities, in partnership with local authorities,
• Contributing to wellbeing and sustainable community development, in partnership with local authorities;
• Protecting health including through a robust system of emergency planning.

Following the implementation of the Health and Social Care Act 2012, local authorities were given new duties to improve the health of their populations (section 12), backed by a ring-fenced grant and a public health team. Local government was to appoint an officer responsible for the new public health function (the director of public health [DPH]) (section 30).

Interviewees and focus group participants in the study commented on changing notions of stewardship, the complexity of governance for public health, ways in which governance failure could be conceptualised, and enablers for the health and wellbeing agenda. While stewardship of the health of the population was considered a key principle of governance, national focus group participants, in particular, described how notions of stewardship were changing from a top-down, collective approach to one based on individual choice (Marks et al.,

2010). This change could be tracked through the increasing influence of the personalisation agenda in health and social care, a movement towards de-professionalisation combined with more local engagement, initiatives for incentivising individual behaviour change and the use of social marketing techniques. However, tensions remained over the balance to be adopted between individualised and collective approaches, and this was key to understanding governance of public health:

> 'The core of what public health faces ... is how much we emphasise the collective over the individual, how much the collective becomes the aggregate of individual decisions, rather than collective decisions imposing individual behaviour.' (National focus group in Marks et al., 2010: 58)

A further issue was a downstream approach to public health while a stewardship role was essentially forward thinking. One focus group participant noted:

> 'The implicit model is we will allow unhealthy social systems to generate disease, but buy it back at the cost of a public health programme. And of course you never get out of that cycle ... and then efficiency in public health is seeing how quickly can we buy this back, what we've just lost, through a decision not taken here, or a view not balanced there.' (Regional focus group in Marks et al., 2010: 57)

There were related concerns over a lack of 'due diligence' in acting on emerging public health hazards:

> 'And that's the bit of public health that's been consistently lost, despite the fact that from what we know had we addressed alcohol, five to ten years ago, we would not be in the position we are now, having lost all the gains from the clinical investment.' (Regional focus group)

Despite these governance concerns expressed by focus group participants, stewardship of the health of the population was described by some PCT interviewees as the raison d'être of their organisation, the 'entire business of the PCT', embedded throughout the commissioning cycle and reflected in investment priorities, in partnership work and in decision-making processes. Governance was about ensuring that processes were in place to link local health needs assessments with strategic development, which in turn should be aligned with financial investment and the achievement of agreed outcomes. These would be reflected in governance processes within the organisation, including the management of provider performance:

> 'The stewardship lies with NHS ... which is what we are, and we have to make sure that our information, our planning, our strategy is absolutely geared into delivering that, and that the contracts and the things that we buy and the supplies and the services that we purchase, etc, and that our suppliers deliver on that, absolutely. The stewardship is a really essential role, and I feel very responsible in terms of carrying a weight of that going forward.' (PCT board chair, site 9)

For PCT interviewees, the stewardship role was often associated with the effective and systematic implementation of the commissioning cycle (further discussed in Chapter Three), although economic stringency could lead to a narrowing of focus and could influence how this role was understood. Practice-based commissioners (PBCs) were more likely to focus on providing continuity in primary care, financial stewardship and ensuring a stable local health economy. It was argued by some interviewees that their training predisposed GPs to focus on individual needs rather than on population health or wider determinants of health, or even on maximising health gain for their practice populations, whether as commissioners or providers. This was reinforced by the payment system for general practice. One PBC lead commented:

> 'Do they have access to the necessary public health skills? Are they going to take responsibility for the whole population and health improvement across the whole population and the partnership work that that engenders and particularly in relation to the wider determinants of health? And I think when you set it up like that the answer's no. They don't have the skills, they don't have the time, they don't have the leadership and they don't really have the will.' (Site 9)

Moreover, while financial balance was recognised as important, the stewardship role for clinicians was focused on the needs of individual patients, described by one professional executive committee (PEC) chair as follows:

'So the financial balance, I understand why the government needs it to be the "be all and end all", but it's not the "be all and end all" for clinicians by any means; being able to improve the lot for our patients is the most important thing.' (PEC chair, site 10)

It was argued that practices still largely thought of themselves as providers wanting 'freedom and flexibilities' and new business opportunities. As health care demands of general practice had expanded, GPs needed to be highly motivated to focus on prevention. A director of finance noted:

'They know that there are all these things that cause ill health but actually they're paid primarily to be a general practitioner. So unless they're really motivated to take time away from treating patients to go and do some of the other stuff, and they'd have to be really motivated to do that. They get well paid for treating patients.' (Site 2)

For interviewees from the voluntary and community sector (VCS), the stewardship role was reflected in their engagement with the grassroots, focusing on the needs of underserved groups and providing a voice for local communities.

Governance arrangements

Governance arrangements cover a wide range of instruments intended to promote accountability and the effective achievement of goals. They can include legal frameworks, policies, incentive structures and a range of audit, scrutiny and performance management arrangements, including targets. Governance arrangements for health, for example, can include public health laws, health-related regulation and audit, health and health care policy implementation, and assessments of the impact of wider policy development on health and health equity. The form these arrangements take, and the balance adopted across regulatory and other approaches, is influenced by the political context. For example, while public health law is applied to infectious disease control and environmental standards, the extent to which it is used to influence risk factors (such as smoking and alcohol) through advertising and marketing restrictions or through taxation and pricing policies will vary with the government in power. Drawing on the Welsh consultation on public health law (Welsh Government, 2012), Galbraith-Emami (2013) reviewed four potential routes (and national examples) for legislation: requirement for health impact assessments across organisations and authorities; imposing statutory duties to reduce inequalities; legislation for a renewed focus on prevention across sectors; and legislation to improve community action around health protection and health improvement.

Developing accountability for health and health equity

Accountability is considered intrinsic to governance, which involves being assured that arrangements are in place, for 'holding to account' those to whom responsibilities have been given who, in turn, have to 'give an account'. In common with governance, the concept is multidimensional and open to multiple interpretations. Accountability can be understood as a principle of governance associated with overlapping principles of transparency and standards of individual conduct; as a particular type of accountability (democratic, corporate, professional or public); or as the implementation of systematic monitoring procedures, notably arrangements for audit and scrutiny. Accountability may be based on the rule of law (in a hierarchical mode of governance) or, in the context of a market, will be achieved through the contract. Partnerships often involve multiple accountabilities and may include, among others, democratic accountability, shareholder accountability, and horizontal accountability across partnerships combined with vertical accountability of individual partnership members to their respective organisations. In the context of the social determinants of health and health equity, accountability for the human right to health involves a 'whole of government' approach aligned with responsibilities within each sector.

Accountability frameworks combine (and measure) these related concepts in different ways. For example, the 'Global accountability framework', developed through One World Trust (Blagescu et al., 2005), integrates into policies, procedures and practice four key dimensions of accountability: transparency; participation; evaluation; and complaint and response mechanisms. Drawing on generic approaches to assessing accountability frameworks (Bovens, 2010), Box 2.1 illustrates their relevance for addressing health and health equity. Questions are reproduced from a wider review of accountability for social determinants of health equity (Marks, in press), where a more detailed account can be found.

Box 2.1: Developing accountability for health and health equity

How is accountability for health and health equity reflected in policy and policy implementation?

Responsibilities for public health need to be made explicit and reflected in statements of accountability not just at a national, political level but across different levels of governance and different organisations (public, private and voluntary). An account of how such responsibilities have been carried out at local, regional and national levels should be provided. There is, for example, a stated commitment to health equity at national level and across sectors in Scotland (Scottish Government, 2008), Finland (Ministry of Social Affairs and Health, 2008), Norway (Ministry of Health and Care Services, 2011) and Sweden (Lundgren, 2009).

How are health inequalities being defined and objectives set; how is progress measured and monitored; and how is information to be communicated to the public, regulators and other stakeholders?

This involves clarifying the various approaches to health equity, such as narrowing the health gap, addressing the social gradient in health, or focusing on disadvantaged groups (Graham, 2009) as each has different policy implications. It means ensuring that relevant data for assessing health equity are collected, analysed and monitored. It is important that data are shared across partners in the interests of joint accountability for shared outcomes.

How is a concern with health and health equity included in the law, incorporated into professional codes of conduct and reflected in decision-making processes?

This can be assessed, for example, through identifying the extent to which health and health equity is reflected in decision making and priority-setting processes (see Chapter Six).

What is the nature of public health 'account giving' (such as reporting mechanisms and public communication strategies)?

Independent public health reports provide one mechanism for account giving related to public health and health equity for a local population, while independent reports of the Chief Medical Officer in England fulfil the same function at a national level. At the time of the study, PCTs were required to publish a prospectus which set out unmet needs, gaps and service priorities and proposals.

What are the systems and levers for holding to account for improved health outcomes?

Levers include performance management arrangements and incentive structures, including arrangements for scrutiny (including local public scrutiny), steering instruments, such as standards and targets, audit and monitoring systems and formal systems for regulation. For health inequalities, there may be national targets (as in England, from 2002-2010) which are monitored, reported on and reflected in implementation strategies and performance management arrangements at local and regional levels. These are further discussed in Chapter Four.

How effective are these systems in identifying failures in responsibility or inadequate control mechanisms? Are they also used for evaluation, research, continuing improvement and for greater policy effectiveness?
A broad and proactive approach to accountability emphasises its potential as an improvement process.

On what basis is the account adjudicated? How is success or failure measured and can appropriate sanctions or complaints procedures be put in place?
For complex public health issues, this aspect of accountability can prove difficult to assess as there is dispersed accountability across sectors and outcomes are both long-term and influenced by many different factors. Moreover, fluctuating approaches to the boundaries of individual and government responsibility, combined with variation in notions of stewardship and state intervention, influence the nature and deployment of sanctions.

Source: The author is grateful to the World Health Organization (WHO) Regional Office for Europe for permission to draw on 'Explanatory note on accountability for social determinants of health equity' a think piece commissioned by the Regional Office for Europe for inclusion in: *Governance for social determinants and equity in health. Companion resource guide. Main principles, current trends and promising practices* (Copenhagen: WHO Regional Office for Europe [in press]).

Accountability for reducing health inequalities should be integrated into governance arrangements and reflected in a coherent approach to regulatory frameworks, targets, monitoring and performance management arrangements. Norway's Public Health Act (Ministry of Health and Care Services, 2011) provides just such a legal framework for holding other sectors accountable for the impact of policies and investments on social inequities (see Box 2.2).

Box 2.2: Norway's Public Health Act

Norway's Public Health Act was intended to 'contribute to societal development that promotes public health and reduces social inequalities in health'. It works through the municipalities which are required to work together and coordinate public health work. Based on a 'whole of government' approach to health and not just on the health sector, it is based on five fundamental principles to underpin policy and action:

- health equity and levelling up the gradient;
- health in all policies, joined-up governance and intersectoral action;
- sustainable development and a long-term perspective;
- precautionary principle: if there is risk of harm do not postpone action because of a lack of scientific consensus;
- participation with multiple stakeholders.

As mentioned earlier, 'holding to account' for addressing complex public health challenges, such as obesity or health inequalities, has proved difficult to achieve: accountability implies both being responsible and having the capacity to control, while accountability for public health is both elusive and dispersed, made more complex by the cumulative and long-term effects of social factors on health. A focus group participant noted that:

> 'There's something about helping people be much clearer about what they can control and deliver locally, and will be held to account for, and what they can do to advocate the change nationally, and how they should work with the public. And I just wonder whether sometimes we haven't really articulated it well enough for people to be held to account, it's been fudged so much that it's almost a smokescreen from actually doing very much.' (Marks et al., 2010: 56)

Accountability for implementing National Institute for Health and Care Excellence (NICE) public health guidance, for example, was difficult to specify. At the time of the study, the Department of Health at central and regional levels, major regulators and NHS boards all shared accountability, power and authority (NHS National Leadership Council, 2010), and PCTs were directly accountable to the Department of Health via Strategic Health Authorities.

The need for more effective processes for public accountability in relation to public health was emphasised in the study, particularly on the part of members of the VCS and of local authority scrutiny committees and board chairs.

> 'But I suppose a really good governance success would be if people felt that they understood how the PCT was spending its resources ... I mean actually wanted to engage with us on particular aspects of the public health agenda.' (PCT board chair, site 1)

VCS members of partnerships considered that their accountability to the public was achieved through their networks and, as one interviewee commented, the VCS were accountable through their membership and governance structures:

> 'I think one of the things that the voluntary sector has got by dint of its structure ... every charity has a governing body, a board, which is made up of voluntary trustees, that's why it's the voluntary sector, so you've got people who are drawn from local communities who are, if you like, in charge of these organisations and if boards are functioning properly that's where a great deal of your public accountability comes from.' (VCS member, site 8)

They argued that there should be greater involvement of the public and the VCS in commissioning for public health outcomes; more transparency in the decision-making processes adopted by commissioners; and a more proactive approach to scrutiny. This reflected the emphasis in commissioning (Department of Health, 2007a) on effective 'voice mechanisms' and community engagement, although, as discussed in Chapter Seven, these were often considered ineffective.

While the Health and Social Care Act 2012 was intended to increase the autonomy of NHS organisations and enhance local accountability, the accountability framework has arguably become more complex. clinical commissioning groups (CCGs) are subject to multiple and overlapping accountabilities – to NHS England, to the public and to statutory health and wellbeing boards (HWBs) – but NHS England excepted, there are limited sanctions in place (Checkland et al., 2013). Providers of NHS services are held accountable through contracts with CCGs. With the transfer of public health responsibilities to local authorities, commissioning for health and wellbeing moved from a context of managerial accountability to one of local democratic accountability, and instead of being a statutory executive member of a PCT board, DsPH became employees of the council (with policy decided by elected councillors). The capacity of local authorities (and of HWBs) to influence CCG commissioning decisions remains unclear, while the relationships between the different (and sometimes overlapping) routes for achieving accountability to the public, including local Healthwatch, lay members of CCG governing bodies, the Cabinet and committees of the local authority, such as the overview and scrutiny committee (OSC), and VCS members of partnership groups, are potentially complex. While the system of targets has been discarded, a main purpose of the public health outcomes framework is 'to provide a framework for transparency and accountability across the public health system' (Department of Health, 2012a: para. 4.1). The extent to which commissioning decisions will be influenced by this outcomes framework remains to be seen.

Modes of governance

Modes of governance include rigid and hierarchical chains of command, loose networks, and markets, where legitimacy is achieved through contracts. Gray (2004), for example, distinguishes between three 'ideal types' of governance: a 'command' mode delivered through hierarchies based on regulatory mechanisms; a 'communion' mode, based on cooperation, trust and common values (a form that is more flexible and adaptable than hierarchies); and a 'contract' mode. 'Command and control' management techniques, for example, are not best suited to complex systems, where flexibility, innovation and local problem solving are needed. In a different classification, Newman adds a self-governance model, reflecting interdependence and reciprocity (Newman, 2001, quoted in Davies et al., 2005: 85) and maps different modes of governance according to their relationship to decentralisation/centralisation and their capacity for continuity/ innovation. Different modes of governance, including the degree of regulation and the flexibility of approaches to implementation, influence 'steering instruments' including incentives (Treib et al., 2005). Debates over the balance to be achieved across individualised and 'solidaristic' incentives across a health system were reflected in the use of incentives to encourage the provision of preventive services, further discussed in Chapter Five.

While there may be broad agreement over underlying principles of governance described earlier, there is far greater debate over the effectiveness of these different modes of governance, how they are reflected across public services as a whole or within specific organisations, the 'mix' that obtains at any one time and how they influence outcomes. In practice, local flexibility, central control and regulation often coexist, reflecting the notion of 'soft bureaucracies' (Courpasson, 2000; Flynn, 2004). Treib et al. (2005) also argue that, in practice, each form of governance may incorporate others, so that, for example, contracts may exist within hierarchical structures. A tripartite categorisation into markets, hierarchies and networks is, therefore, considered too simplistic given these hybrid, or mixed, forms of governance which coexist within publicly funded services.

The extent to which the state moves away from direct control towards regulation is a further key governance issue, often categorised as the shift from 'government' to 'governance'. Self organising interorganisational networks have been described as becoming 'increasingly prominent among British governing structures' (Rhodes, 1996: 658), complementing markets and hierarchies. The phrase 'new modes of governance' has been used to encapsulate this variety of networked approaches (Weale, 2011), although it has also been pointed out that networks are hardly a new organisational form (Goodwin et al., 2004). It has also been argued that the shift from government to governance (and therefore to a network mode of governance) has been greatly exaggerated (Davies, 2011) and that hierarchical forms of governance continue to dominate.

The complex mix of governance arrangements within the NHS has been interpreted within the framework of 'new public management' (NPM), associated with a realignment of the role of the state, moving away from traditional bureaucracies to combinations of 'targets and markets', where performance is controlled by a combination of state control via performance management regimes, and choice and competition from outside (Cooke and Muir, 2012). Davies et al. (2005: 82) summarise changes commonly subsumed under NPM as:

> a strong emphasis on efficiency savings, meeting performance targets, private sector freedom to manage, regulation, and restructuring to introduce quasi markets and to create more autonomous agencies.

NPM has been criticised for its intraorganisational focus and inability to make links or preserve trust across organisations, or to negotiate complex accountabilities across them (Rhodes, 1996). Also, as Saltman (2002: 1682) comments, the complexity of exercising authority through oversight of markets rather than through 'command and control' should not be underestimated:

Negotiating and monitoring contracts is more complicated and personnel intensive than paying a budget; designing outcome tied regulations is more complicated than issuing rules and circulars.

Elements of NPM are reflected in the current health system in England, with its increased emphasis on separating commissioners from providers, encouraging greater plurality of providers, including the private sector, and promoting a degree of autonomy within a national system which sets standards and monitors through independent systems of regulation. The NHS has been described as a combination, from its inception, of quasi-hierarchy, quasi-markets and quasi-networks (Exworthy et al., 1999), although, unlike Scotland and Wales, the NHS reform programme in England has increasingly embraced elements of the market. In particular, private sector provision of NHS-funded care has been encouraged under the coalition government, despite evidence that an internal market in health care neither promotes efficiency nor furthers the principle of social justice (Hunter, 2013). More emphasis has been placed on competition (through policies on patient choice, payment by results and a plurality of providers) than on integration and collaboration (Ham, 2007). Networks, although widespread in the NHS, are not fully self-organising and work within national directives. The NHS remains a largely centralised system with national priorities and assessments of standards through independent regulatory agencies, such as Monitor and the Care Quality Commission (CQC). In a study of governance mechanisms in commissioning and providing hospital, community and GP-based health care (from 1991 to 2005), for example, Abbott (2006: 15) showed that the dominant strategic governance mechanism was 'upward hierarchical accountability to national government', although there was evidence of markets and networks at a tactical level. He argues that reducing layers between central government and frontline services, a process often described as the 'hollowing out of the state', had instead served to increase 'centralised direction'.

The coexistence of market, network and hierarchical modes of governance within the NHS is associated with tensions arising from inherent contradictions between cooperation and competition; the difficulties of integrating services at the same time as promoting a competitive market; and potential conflicts of interest for those who concurrently commission and provide services. (This was the case with PBC at the time of the study and continues from April 2013, through CCGs). Commissioners also have to be aware of the potential for market failure. A market mode of governance works against partnership working and collaborative commissioning, which are key for integrating health and social care, addressing long-term conditions and for working across sectors in promoting population health. Partnership working is also important in order to limit 'risk shunting' across commissioners and providers, and 'cost shunting' across different parts of a local health system.

Partnership governance, an example of networked governance, is discussed in more detail in the following section and illustrated with views from the study at a time when the number of partnerships escalated and partnership working across a local area became a policy requirement.

Partnership governance

Working through partnerships and networks across a local area – spanning health, local authorities, the VCS and the private sector – and across sectors at a national level has been considered key for addressing wider determinants of health and health equity, although evidence of the effectiveness of partnerships in improving health outcomes remains elusive (Perkins et al., 2010). *Strong and prosperous communities: The local government White Paper* (Secretary of State for Communities and Local Government, 2006) drew attention to the importance of partnership in public health, calling for 'more visible local leadership for health and wellbeing' (p. 14), joined-up performance management and 'greater clarity' over agreeing and delivering local health and wellbeing targets. While partnerships were seen as a means for fostering devolved solutions to local problems, the extent to which they were able to depart from national policies was, nevertheless, limited (Improvement and Development Agency, 2007).

While local partnerships have been established for commissioning and delivering specific preventive services which span different organisations (as is the case, for example, for aspects of sexual health services, lifestyle interventions and drug and alcohol services), difficulties in achieving partnership working, whether at national or local level (or across different levels of governance) have been documented for public health (Hunter and Perkins, 2014) and, in particular, for health and social care partnerships (Glasby and Dickinson, 2014). Difficulties at local level are replicated at national level: a report from the Institute for Government (Gash et al., 2008: 10) noted that:

Incentives for Whitehall to work cross departmentally remain weak. There is virtually no pooling of resources to support cross departmental policies despite the fact that central government itself recognises that such pooling is a powerful incentive for partners to work collectively and to make the necessary trade-offs between conflicting priorities.

In response to these problems, a range of partnership governance frameworks and 'toolkits' have been developed (Audit Commission, 2007) and it is recognised that partnerships need well developed performance management arrangements in order to succeed (Audit Commission, 2009a). Partnerships involve risks as well as benefits: both need to be identified in advance. Building trust can be time consuming, there may be conflicting goals, values or ways of working, and individual members may have differing capacities to influence decision making in the partnership or in their respective organisations. A report on NHS board governance (NHS National Leadership Council, 2010) highlighted the importance of partnership agreements, clear perspectives on care pathways, transparency of strategic decision making and clarity of outcomes. All of these needed to be reflected in arrangements for reporting and monitoring performance, managing risk and ensuring accountability.

Different types of accountability coexist in partnerships and these are a source of governance tension. Public health inevitably involves working across different sectors in complex partnership arrangements with multiple accountabilities, where success is dependent on building coalitions. There are lines of accountability to the respective organisations making up the partnership, at the same time as horizontal accountability for achieving shared partnership-wide objectives. Local authorities also have a democratic mandate while community participants seek to reflect the local VCS, itself diverse, and there are complex arrangements across the various themed subgroups of local partnerships. Where accountability mechanisms remain unclear it will be difficult to hold partnerships to account. Tuohy (2003: 202), for example, writes of the need for a 'new governance paradigm' to 'connote the processes and instruments of governing in the context of complex organisational networks in which no one set of actors has the authority to "command and control"'. The development of partnership-wide accountability frameworks which include clarity over the rationale of the partnership, decision-making roles of partnership members in their respective organisations and agreements over financial and risk management may help to overcome 'silo working' in partnerships, identify contradictory incentives and promote adoption of partnership over single organisation goals (Audit Commission, 2005). However, devolved solutions have been hampered by organisational and financial barriers.

Partnership working was promoted throughout the period of the Labour government: at the time of the study, this was reflected in performance management arrangements, including the world class commissioning (WCC) assurance process and the comprehensive area assessment (CAA) carried out across a local authority area and specifically designed to assess the extent to which partners worked together to improve outcomes. These were all considered by interviewees in the study as encouraging partnerships for health and wellbeing. Partnerships were considered key for agreeing and monitoring local area agreements (LAAs) across a local authority area. Partnership working was also reflected in national policy initiatives for joint working such as 'Total Place', a whole-area approach to local public services (HM Treasury and Department for Communities and Local Government, 2010), integrated care pilots and integrated working under the aegis of statutory Children's Trusts (which were later reshaped by the coalition government).

Local strategic partnerships (LSPs) (around 360 were in place across England at the time of the study) and their themed subgroups were the focus for local health partnerships. They were responsible for delivery of a Sustainable Community Strategy, which all local authorities had to produce (a requirement subsequently abolished by the coalition government). Covering a local authority area, LSPs were described as a key governance structure 'highlighting and resolving cross-departmental and cross-agency conflicts' (Gash et al., 2008: 8). They were not statutory organisations and therefore not subject to statutory reporting or inspection regimes (although there was a statutory duty of partnership). Despite the original intention that LSPs would simplify local partnerships, there were concerns over their accountability arrangements, over governance across the partnership and their capacity to fufil the demands made of them. There was also evidence of poor links with neighbourhoods (White et al., 2006). There were complex accountability arrangements between LSPs and local authorities, and between VCS members of LSPs and the organisations or community networks they represented. Cutting across these organisational accountabilities were tensions between participatory styles of decision making and accountability based on local democracy (Marks, 2007). These difficulties were compounded by the creation of performance management systems which undermined local priority setting and concerns over the effects on local engagement if commissioners focused on performance management systems linked to national targets.

Views of partnership in the study

Focus group participants and interviewees considered partnership arrangements a key area of concern for public health. All groups of interviewees recognised that promoting health and wellbeing required working across agencies to address the wider determinants of health and that partnerships played an important role in improving health outcomes over the longer term:

> 'And there's issues around improving lifestyles which will help in the shorter term and that's partly within the gift of the health services and partly within the gift of partners.... As you get into the longer term, it's around working with local authorities to get regeneration into there and get employment opportunities, improve educational attainment, get the right kind of levels of training and education for people to take the jobs that would come into the area. Now we're working in all those areas through the county council but that doesn't exclude the need to address the people where the harm's already been done now.' (DPH, site 9)

Numerous initiatives had emerged from local partnerships, including weight management and smoking cessation services; shared funding; joint posts for developing local neighbourhood approaches; healthy lifestyle managers working with PBC consortia; health trainers and free swimming.

The extent of partnership working for health and wellbeing could be gauged through a number of routes. As discussed further in Chapter Three, one aspect was the 'jointness' of the joint strategic needs assessment (JSNA), but there were many other examples, such as joint scenario modelling to gauge future health needs; alignment of third sector commissioning strategies across PCTs and local authorities; pooled budgets and joint posts; the inclusion of local authorities in care pathway development; and shared approaches to performance management. It was argued that much could be achieved through aligning budgets, thereby avoiding complex governance arrangements required in order to formally pool budgets, but clear governance arrangements were necessary.

Focus groups and interviewees discussed partnership governance, including different ways of monitoring and evaluating initiatives across partnerships, ensuring that governance between organisations met agreed criteria and creating clear accountability arrangements. However, there were inevitably differences in culture and procedures between organisations. It was argued that governance arrangements for partnerships lacked clarity, given different systems of regulation across PCTs and local authorities, and that public health targets were less rigorously monitored in the latter. At a local level, it was important to develop a collaborative approach across the system, ensuring that LAAs and the NHS Annual Operating Plans were jointly considered.

One of the major barriers to partnership working was the emphasis on 'single organisational success', which was reinforced in governance mechanisms.

> 'I mean part of the issue why systems don't deliver what the aspirations are is because the reward systems are not aligned to the behaviours we want in the system. If you look at the reward systems for civil servants, it's having your own area, it being important and you delivering that upon that area. It's not for spending 10% of your time working with someone else on their area, you know what I mean, it's not what the system's rewarding.' (National focus group in Marks et al., 2010: 57)

Governance structures for health and wellbeing were unclear at the interfaces of interagency working:

> 'But actually, you know, when it comes down to the interagency bit, all those systems seem to collapse.... And that seems to me the territory that public health is in, you know, that's where public health governance is, and actually we haven't solved the governance system there.' (National focus group in Marks et al., 2010: 56)

While PCT interviewees generally viewed PCT governance mechanisms as robust, partnership governance was considered less well developed:

> 'But there's also I think big questions around integrated and partnership governance, ... where we're making joint investments in quite a lot of things. I'm thinking around

children's services as a for instance. That currently as I said earlier is tracked separately through our own boards and through our own corporations ... there's a kind of issue around satisfying and continuing to satisfy our own organisations and the regulatory bodies that currently exist but also doing it also in a more integrated way.' (PCT chair, site 9)

A chief executive went further in his criticisms of partnership governance, highlighting the failure to link partnership decisions to those made by organisations represented in the partnership:

'I've never yet seen an organisation that can list all its staff that attend the relevant, even the statutory partnerships, that if a partnership agrees the strategy do they then work out the implications for each organisation? Does that implication get communicated back to the organisation.... Having agreed it how do others then hold them to account? And if you're running a shared target through it how do we hold somebody else to account for their bit? And I've never yet come across anyone or any place that can give me clear answers to those sorts of questions, so I think there is a major weakness about this, about partnership governance that needs to be better addressed than it is at the moment.' (Site 3)

Accountability arrangements between partnerships and their subgroups could also create difficulties. While health partnerships had developed terms of reference for working within their partnership with accountability to the LSP, links between subgroups did not reflect the cross-cutting nature of the health and wellbeing agenda. Concerns were expressed by VCS interviewees in all the case study sites that themed partnerships under the LSP worked against a whole-system approach.

One of the consequences of governance complexity was an emphasis on the role of local leaders with skills to understand and negotiate a wide range of governance arrangements. However, a number of barriers to effective partnership working for health and wellbeing were also identified. First was the breadth of the health and wellbeing agenda, which made it difficult to engage, as one interviewee noted:

'Because certainly the discussions we've had at local strategic partnership level has been actually health and wellbeing is so all encompassing that there's a tendency for everybody to go "It's not my problem."' (Director of strategy, site 3)

Second, partnerships and governance arrangements were prey to constant change through reorganisations, 'fiddling around with the boundaries', or as a result of shifts in the political agenda. A PEC chair commented:

> 'And every time you have a shift of structure, you have to reorganise your governance structures, which potentially undermines those structures. Because governance is around having a clear idea of what you're measuring, how you're measuring it, and making sure it's safe and effective. You get that in place and then say oh no, no, we're reorganising it all.... So I think every time you have a reorganisation or a restructure, not that they shouldn't happen, I think it potentially undermines governance for some length of time.' (Site 5)

Moreover, the reorganisation of PCTs in 2006 (reducing their numbers from 303 to 152) had led to a loss of locality focus which was considered a retrograde step, breaking up partnerships and making it more difficult to link into neighbourhood management structures.

Third were problems of coterminosity. A lack of coterminosity across PCTs and local authorities, and multiple partnerships spanning different boundaries could lead to a lack of capacity to engage. This created problems in aligning priorities, providing input and manpower to local partnerships, especially in areas with numerous district councils, or supporting LAAs across different councils. OSCs struggled to engage all the stakeholders across such a wide area and the VCS described difficulties in coordinating their work across large geographical areas. Resources to cover the costs of VCS involvement were limited and the lack of an umbrella VCS body could make it difficult to coordinate views.

Fourth were perceptions over unequal status of the VCS, even though partnerships were potentially an effective route for greater engagement. In four sites, interviewees from the VCS expressed the view that engagement in partnerships was tokenistic, as one interviewee commented:

> 'The VCS is often seen as a kind of poorer partner, you know, we need to feel privileged to be able to get at the

LIBRARY, UNIVERSITY OF CHESTER

table. Well that's not the right approach and actually it should be what we can learn from each other.' (Site 3)

This could mean that the local VCS was not linked into wider partnership strategies and targets, although this problem could partly be overcome by overarching bodies which could gather views of local VCS organisations:

'I'd definitely like to see more of the third sector organisations' experiences and, if you like, intelligence in terms of what they are involved in delivering. I'd like to see that communicated again more systematically to health commissioners so that they can use that information to inform their commissioning choices.' (VCS member, site 8)

Finally, financial pressures put partnerships under strain:

'But inevitably when the pressure's on financially, they [the organisational boundaries] get in the way, so you know you get the whole cost shunting debate, with health shunting cost to social care, or social care shunting cost to health.' (Director of strategic commissioning, site 10)

The importance of building coalitions across partnerships which reflected different motivations, interests and accountabilities was reflected in expectations of public health leadership. Most of the DsPH in the study were joint appointments across the PCT and the local authority, but were accountable to the PCT. Local authorities had a democratic mandate, which was lacking in PCTs and this created ambiguities over public health leadership. Although joint appointments were perceived as routes for attempting to bridge the organisational and cultural divide, the dispersal of a public health agenda across different departments, partnerships and subgroups created problems.

'Things that influence public health that are within the remit of the local authority are actually spread throughout the structure of the local authority, so there's no one bit of the local authority that does public health because everything, from housing, transport, economic policy, parks and countryside, children and young people services, adult social services, I mean you name it, it all has an impact, one way or another, on public health.... But because it's not

brought together and focused in one place it's very difficult
to get a handle on it all.' (DPH, site 7)

Moreover, there was a contrast between a PCT agenda, largely focused
on behaviour change and promoting healthy lifestyles, and an emphasis
in local authorities on assessing health impact of local policies and
promoting social and environmental change. Differences in culture
and in accountability arrangements, combined with the breadth of a
public health agenda, created challenges for partnership governance.
This was sometimes reflected in 'silo working' in public health and a
lack of integration across multi-agency structures.

Although the commissioning landscape has changed since 2013,
with the abolition of PCTs and the creation of CCGs and HWBs,
tensions associated with partnership governance are likely to persist. A
review of HWBs 'one year on' (Humphries and Galea, 2013) showed
good progress in establishing the boards but some familiar concerns
were raised: despite a 'rhetoric of localism' there were concerns over
whether local priorities would prevail in practice; partner organisations
had different measures of success; and the new NHS organisational
structures were complex with some ambiguity in accountability
arrangements. For example, members of CCGs are accountable for
partnership decisions (though their membership of the HWB), to
their own decision-making CCG boards, to NHS England and to
local populations.

Most often cited, however, was the financial climate and, as discussed
earlier, this raises risks of cost shunting across organisations. The review
pointed out that few boards cited public engagement as a priority, and
this reflects views in the study of a tokenistic approach to the VCS. As
with LSPs and PCTs, lack of coterminosity continues to be a problem.
Finally, HWBs are not decision-making bodies and they lack funds
or formal powers to influence commissioning decisions. Much will
therefore depend on their capacity to influence through partnership.

Levels of governance

While governance arrangements can be considered at each level of
organisation (national, local or regional), they increasingly operate
internationally. Hooghe and Marks (2001) note the development
of different tiers of governance and a range of new phrases to suit,
for example, 'multilevel governance', 'multi-tiered governance',
'polycentric governance' and 'multi-perspectival governance'. They
comment that these different 'levels' of governance, ranging from EU

directives and incentives to partnerships at subregional and community levels, interrelate in different ways, adding a further complexity to collaboration within any single forum or across different geographical areas. Public health challenges are made more complex by the impact of multilevel governance, including the influence of the EU and other international decision-making bodies. In a study of multilevel governance in England, Townsend (2005) documents the different levels of governance that have been instituted 'at different dates and for different purposes', commenting on the complex and sometimes ambiguous accountability arrangements which emerge, and the capacity for 'jumping' across different layers of governance. He argues that working across institutional boundaries through personal networks is an important indicator of success in negotiating the complexities of multilevel governance. In the same vein, it has been argued that 'strategic systems leadership', involving less top-down or directive approaches, forms a more appropriate response to complex policy issues (Hallsworth, 2011).

The example of corporate governance

At a corporate level, governance encompasses the processes, policies and laws affecting the ways in which corporations are controlled, and managers and others, including different professions, are held to account. The Audit Commission (2003: 4) for example, defined corporate governance as:

> the framework of accountability to users, stakeholders and the wider community, within which organisations take decisions, and lead and control their functions, to achieve their objectives.

Effective corporate governance combines 'hard' factors (that is, systems and processes for the management of risk, finance and performance) with 'soft' factors, including leadership, integrity and standards of behaviour (Audit Commission, 2003). Corporate governance arrangements are intended to support effective decision making within a clear framework of accountability, in line with underlying principles and national standards. For NHS organisations, these underlying values are reflected in the NHS Constitution (Department of Health, 2013b). NHS boards need to ensure that principles of governance (such as transparency and accountability) are upheld and that the underlying values of the organisation are reflected in governance structures related to financial stewardship, risk management (financial, corporate and clinical), audit, information, clinical governance and service quality. In the study, PCT interviewees interpreted governance as mainly corporate governance:

> 'I mean my understanding, I always struggle a bit with governance, exactly what it means, is that there is good oversight of the purpose, aims, systems and processes which are in place to deliver that, and that is monitored to show that it is being done to best effect with the best possible outcomes.' (Director of strategy, site 2)

From a corporate perspective, effective governance was often associated with compliance with national standards, public accountability and with having a clear idea of the organisation's purpose and what was required for achieving its aims. For example, implementation of health care standards was seen as a route for demonstrating effective governance in PCTs at the time of the study:

> 'You can demonstrate effective governance through the application of Healthcare Commission standards. So if you're applying appropriate public health standards which apply to all NHS bodies, then you can demonstrate good governance.' (DPH, site 6)

In the study, PCT interviewees often identified good governance with effective organisational governance. From this perspective, public health governance was embedded in the governance arrangements of the organisation. In line with this, the concept of 'public health governance' was questioned by a number of interviewees:

> 'Well no, I think the phrase is unhelpful – public health governance. I think it is because in PCTs you have an integrated governance approach, you know, so you have integrated systems of direction and control, and dependent on what it is certain people either lead it or control it or monitor it or assure it.' (Deputy chief executive, site 8)

The identification of governance with corporate governance meant that there was less discussion by PCT interviewees than by focus group participants about the governance implications of working across a local public health system.

Towards governance for health

Governance for population health involves understanding the impact of different dimensions of governance and negotiating complex governance arrangements across partnerships, networks and sectors. As Table 2.1 shows, the range of governance dimensions can be applied to specific topic areas such as climate change or digital governance. In the NHS, for example, the concept of clinical governance is well developed, in stark contrast to what could be considered a complementary concept of public health governance. This is in spite of PCTs having responsibility for improving health and tackling health inequalities at the time of the study. Clinical governance is an umbrella term covering audit, risk management, quality assurance and continuous quality improvement, and is reflected in professional performance, resource allocation, risk management and patient satisfaction. It has been defined as 'a system through which NHS organisations are accountable for continuously improving the quality of their services and safeguarding high standards of care by creating an environment in which excellence in clinical care will flourish' (Scally and Donaldson, 1998: 62). Governance arrangements related to clinical quality reflect a systematic approach to addressing failure: what is involved in 'public health governance' could be highlighted through a similar systematic approach. How are failures in protecting population health identified, measured and monitored? What arrangements are in place to ensure that population health is continuously improved and health inequalities narrowed?

Despite arguments that clinical governance be incorporated within a system of integrated governance, a report by the Audit Commission (2003) highlighted the existence of separate governance streams for clinical governance and corporate governance in committee structures beneath PCT board level. It concluded that:

> The consequences of this are that the clinical arm of the organisation wants to, and often does, deliver excellent clinical care to some individual patients, but not always with due regard for equity, finance and the bigger community picture. (p. 12)

While their report highlights the importance of combining these streams of governance, it also serves to draw attention to the historical emphasis on clinical governance in the NHS and the neglect of a parallel concept of 'public health governance'. Arguably, the emphasis on clinical governance and its status as a reference point for quality assurance worked against the development of its public health equivalent within the NHS at the time of the study. While there were attempts to streamline assurance frameworks in PCTs (and, in particular, to integrate risk management arrangements), connections were not always made. For example, public health was not considered as a separate governance strand (in contrast to clinical governance) and was poorly integrated with other governance arrangements.

The application to public health of the systematic approach developed for clinical governance was discussed in two case study sites. For example, one interviewee stated:

> 'So it would be quite interesting to, say, take what we apply to clinical governance and debate whether you have the same thing in public health. So do you have people clearly in charge of it, have we got the right training courses so our staff are appropriately skilled, have we got the right processes that will get the right bits of public health in the right order? Does the board pay significant attention, does it receive the appropriate reports at the appropriate time? So it would be quite an interesting line of thought.' (Assistant CE, site 5 in Marks et al., 2011c: 19)

This was reiterated by an interviewee in a different site, who commented:

> 'I think ... something about the failures in public health governance is that for so long public health has just been off the radar that any governance of public health is good because at least it shows that there's something to govern, if you like.' (Director of strategy, site 3)

The complexity of governance arrangements relevant to improving health was a common thread in all three focus groups. It was argued that concentrating on certain aspects of governance could lead to the neglect of others. For example, focusing on organisational governance arrangements within the NHS (as commonly reflected by PCT interviewees) could deflect attention from underlying principles of stewardship across a local public health system. Effective stewardship involved understanding what could be achieved at national, regional or local levels and recognising the breadth of a local public health system, along with the levers for change across the public sector. Participants argued that public health governance should therefore reflect a broader public health system, including social and economic regeneration and social care, rather than be associated with a single professional group or with a specific organisation. One participant noted that:

> 'It is for me also increasingly difficult to talk about public health in isolation from sort of public health and wellbeing and the broader links into local regeneration by social and economic regeneration strategies. And I find it quite artificial to separate it out into a sort of compartment of its own, both at that end but also in terms of its links into social care, care of the disadvantaged too. It's the broader basis.' (National focus group)

This approach would involve identifying how resources could be mobilised across the public sector as a whole and it was argued that current governance arrangements did not enable this level of debate. Public health professionals needed to clarify the health consequences of public policy and economic decision making. This implied holding agencies to account for preventable morbidity and premature mortality across the system.

While clarity over accountability constituted a key dimension of governance, focus group participants also argued that, in practice, accountability for health and wellbeing remained dispersed and ill defined. If complex arrangements were to be successfully negotiated and health integrated into the range of governance structures, effective leadership was required. Accountability arrangements in partnerships were identified as a key aspect of governance rendered more complex by differing accountability arrangements in PCTs and local authorities:

> 'Local authorities have some form of democratic accountability but the lack of clear coordination ... in terms of public health leadership between local authorities and NHS organisations, and PCTs in particular, have meant it is very hard to understand where leadership on a public health agenda is, what communities or local areas are covered and how that actually, you know, is planned, organised and how there's strategic direction.' (Marks et al., 2010: 56–7)

Responsibility was dispersed across agencies and there was a lack of personal accountability for creating a coherent pattern of provision. As mentioned earlier, one of the barriers to partnership working was the emphasis on single organisational success, which was reinforced in governance mechanisms.

Focus group participants highlighted a wide range of 'governance failures', including a lack of clear accountability for the persistence of health inequalities, failure to make the case with the public for investing in public health priorities, and a lack of due diligence and timely action across a public health system on hazards such as alcohol, obesity or debt. Proactive approaches to local environmental risk were needed along with identification of public health consequences of policy decisions and a less narrow approach to the public health evidence base. Performance management arrangements (see Chapter Four) were described as ill-aligned, focused on specific organisations and weighted towards national priorities and targets. A further governance failure was a lack of clarity over how best to coordinate strategies across different agencies.

Conclusions

Studies of governance and of the impact of various modes of governance on health outcomes have often focused on health care services, neglecting the impact on population health. While it is argued that a market mode of governance may promote efficiency, markets do not provide an obvious route for promoting equity. Neither does a focus on consumer (or client) demand lend itself to population-based approaches. An emphasis on choice as a route to improving the quality of services is also likely to increase inequalities, as the capacity to exercise choice is not equally distributed. In addition, the benefits of separating commissioning from providing services, a key element for creating markets in health care, are not evident from the point of view of encouraging partnership working, collaboration across agencies or the integration of services.

Governance arrangements are intended to promote effective decision making in line with the values of an organisation, but a concentration on some aspects of governance may lead to the neglect of others. Where a stewardship role is narrowly defined, public health priorities may not be integrated into board governance arrangements or decision-making processes; where the focus is on governance arrangements within a single organisation, then the concept of stewardship across a wider heath system may be lost. Moreover, the ways in which targets and incentives are structured within performance management systems can work against areas of public health activity with multiple objectives and where outcomes are long term.

In practice, 'good governance' in relation to population health involves an explicit commitment to promoting equity in national strategies and policies, and assessing policies through processes for health (and health inequality) impact assessment. This underlying principle needs to be reflected through intersectoral partnerships and through governance arrangements, such as audit and performance management. The relocation of public health into local authorities is likely to reinvigorate debate over how best to maximise public health benefits through working across the public sector while at the same time encouraging a more participatory approach to public health decision making.

Note
[1] See: http://info.worldbank.org/governance/wgi/index.aspx#home.

CHAPTER THREE

Commissioning for health and wellbeing

Commissioning needs to be more proactive, transformational and forward looking, focusing on promoting good health, investing for prevention, independence and wellbeing. The skills to do this are relatively scarce and require systematic support and development. (Department of Health, 2007a: 15)

'The overall emphasis on commissioning for health and wellbeing I don't think has changed. We just don't have the money to do it with.' (Director of public health [DPH], 2009, site 7)

Commissioning decisions are influenced by each of the governance dimensions outlined in the previous chapter, while the commissioning process itself can provide a route for involving communities and for making services more accountable. The extent to which underlying governance principles, such as social equity or accountability, are reflected in national policies and in governance arrangements will influence decision making at a local level, as will the importance attached nationally to the prevention of ill health. However, even where there is national policy commitment, to social equity for example, this may be imperfectly translated into local practice. There is room for manoeuvre over the relative emphasis accorded to each phase of a commissioning cycle, over the extent to which health equity is built into contracts with providers, over partnership arrangements, the choice of incentives and over deployment of any additional resources. For primary care trusts (PCTs), certain phases of the commissioning cycle predominated, in particular, purchasing or transactional elements and negotiations with providers of acute health care services. This was, in part, a consequence of supply side dominance, the requirement for PCTs to achieve financial balance and an emphasis on acute sector targets in performance management.

This chapter begins by outlining the history of NHS commissioning in England. This originates in policy decisions of Conservative and Labour governments since the 1990s to separate the task of commissioning services from the responsibility for providing them, as a precondition for policies which promoted patient choice and provider diversity as a route to improved quality and efficiency. It then describes the commissioning cycle as promoted under the world class commissioning (WCC) initiative of the Labour government which in theory, if not always in practice, encouraged a public health-led approach to commissioning. Health needs assessment of the population is discussed in some detail as the first stage in a commissioning cycle and as a cornerstone of a public health-led approach to commissioning. This activity is internationally recognised as an 'essential public health operation' (WHO, 2012b) and its status has been enhanced in the NHS reforms of the coalition government. The chapter summarises interviewee views over the role and influence of the joint strategic needs assessment (JSNA), originally introduced in England in 2008. It also discusses the extent to which JSNAs reflected not only the importance of a partnership approach but also partnership tensions. Given current responsibilities of GPs in commissioning through their membership of clinical commissioning groups (CCGs), the chapter discusses the degree of engagement of GP practices with the preventive agenda and with JSNAs in particular. At the time of the study, practice-based commissioning (PBC) was the route through which GPs were intended to engage with commissioning decisions, following the demise of GP fundholding and of Total Purchasing Pilots (discussed in the following section). The chapter then reviews approaches to tackling health inequalities and draws on the study to summarise enablers and barriers for commissioning for health and wellbeing. It concludes by identifying areas of continuity and change following the major changes in commissioning arrangements introduced by the coalition government. Three key aspects of commissioning for health and wellbeing, that is, the use of incentives for preventive services, prioritising investment in prevention and public involvement in commissioning are the subject of Chapters Five to Seven.

Commissioning in England: choice and the market model

Use of the term 'commissioning' is relatively recent but the tasks involved are generic. The Health Committee (House of Commons Health Committee, 2011: para. 2) noted that:

Although the term 'commissioning' has only been in use since the 1990s, the functions it refers to have been present, in one form or another, since the inception of the NHS. It has always been necessary to determine the health needs of the population and to design services accordingly, with due regard to the available level of resources. The NHS has also always aspired to ensure that its services meet high quality standards.

The search for a commissioning function which is clearly separated from providing services has been a consistent theme running through reorganisations of the NHS in England since the 1990s. This separation of commissioning from provision was initiated and pursued through the Conservative government's *Working for patients* reforms (Secretaries of State for Health, Wales, Scotland and Northern Ireland, 1989), implemented from the early 1990s and associated with the encouragement of a market. Over the same period, there were attempts to increase the engagement of GP practices in commissioning, initially through GP fundholding (1991–7), which gave GPs real budgets for commissioning selected services, and subsequently though Total Purchasing Pilots (1994–7), an extended version of fundholding (Mays et al., 1997) which involved GPs in commissioning potentially all health services for a defined population.

The Labour government (1997–2010) retained the purchaser/provider split in its 10-year plan for the English NHS, *The new NHS: Modern, dependable* (Secretary of State for Health, 1997). From 2002, it set in motion a series of market-related reforms spanning patient choice of elective care, 'payment by results' (from 2003/4) (where funding followed the patient, replacing the previous system of block contracts) and encouragement of provider diversity in the NHS, including a greater role for the private sector. These reforms (and subsequent initiatives related to high quality, integrated and personalised care for long-term conditions and improved quality (Secretary of State for Health, 2008; Mays, 2013) were the subject of an extensive Department of Health funded evaluation programme to establish whether intended changes had occurred in practice and to evaluate their impact.[1] The Health Reform Evaluation Programme was largely focused on health care where the effects of the market-related reforms were described as 'mostly modest' (Mays and Tan, 2012). The reforms did not apply in the same way to all areas of care or in all contexts; there were high transaction costs; and there were inconsistencies between different strands of the reforms, as well as between the reforms as a whole and cooperative ways of working already established across commissioners and providers (Frosini et al., 2012).

Encouraging stronger commissioning was a major plank of the reforms and, in 2000, PCTs were reinvented as commissioning organisations (and became fully established in 2002) (Department of Health, 2005). However, the speed at which PCTs separated their commissioning role from their traditional role in directly managing community health services was variable. This was addressed through the NHS operating framework for 2008/9, which required an internal separation and, in 2009, *Transforming community services: Enabling new patterns of provision* (Department of Health, 2009b: 7) made it clear that 'by April 2009 all PCT direct provider organisations should have moved into a contractual relationship with their PCT commissioning function.... This means ensuring sufficient separation of roles within the PCT to avoid direct conflicts of interest.' This separation was not uniformly welcomed by PCTs, given its association with short-term contracts, the potential for fragmentation and a loss of infrastructure. GP fundholding had been rapidly abolished by the incoming Labour government in 1997 (in line with its long-standing opposition to the scheme due to concerns over its divisive nature, impact on equity and transaction costs). PBC was launched from 2005 and was intended to promote the involvement of GPs and other primary care professionals in commissioning and in redesigning services. While PBC consortia were allocated an indicative budget, statutory responsibility remained with PCTs. As for commissioning arrangements, the key development over the period of the study was the ambitious programme for WCC (Department of Health, 2007b). This clarified the purpose of commissioning and the skills required to commission for improved health outcomes. The aims of WCC were to improve population health and address inequalities, 'adding life to years and years to life'. The WCC 'vision' (Department of Health, 2007b: 1) stated that:

> The NHS has real potential to develop world class commissioning – investing NHS funds to secure the maximum improvement in health and wellbeing outcomes from the available resources. As world class commissioners, primary care trusts (PCTs) must take on the mantle of trusted community leaders, working with their local population, partners and clinicians, leading the local NHS.

This programme represented an important shift in emphasis: from commissioning as purchasing of health care services to commissioning as a continuous process, reflected in the phases of a commissioning cycle and linked to an assurance framework.

With the advent of the coalition government in 2010, PCTs were abolished along with the WCC assurance framework. New CCGs, to which all GPs had to belong, were established as statutory organisations with real budgets and as the main commissioners of NHS services. Although the post-Coalition reconfiguration of commissioning has some parallels with the Total Purchasing Pilots of the 1990s, the story of commissioning in England is not one of straightforward evolution but of contested argument, in particular over the implementation and extent of changes designed to ensure competition in providing health care services, the use of the private sector to provide NHS-funded services, and the ways in which GPs can best be encouraged to engage with commissioning. These debates continue to influence the commissioning context and options available to commissioners.

NHS services have been made increasingly open to competition, as reflected in the contested section 75 of the Health and Social Care Act 2012. It was pointed out by numerous commentators (House of Commons Health Committee, 2011; Timmins, 2012) that there had been a major policy shift from *Our programme for government*, published by the coalition government in May 2010 (HM Government, 2010a) to the publication of the White Paper, *Equity and excellence: Liberating the NHS* (Secretary of State for Health, 2010a), just two months later. New plans to abolish PCTs formed part of what the Health Committee described as a 'significant institutional upheaval' set in motion by the White Paper. While aims to improve health and address health inequalities are two of the overarching indicators in the public health and NHS outcomes frameworks (Department of Health, 2012a, 2012b), tensions over optimum population size for commissioning organisations, governance arrangements and priority setting are likely to persist.

The study almost exactly coincided with the period of WCC (2007–10) and of concerted attempts to strengthen the role of PCTs as commissioning organisations. It began in 2007, soon after the publication of the *Commissioning framework for health and well-being* (Department of Health, 2007a). Building on the White Paper, *Our health, our care, our say* (Secretary of State for Health, 2006), this document combined 'vision, framework and practical proposals', where the 'vision' was to move away from a narrow focus on the treatment of ill health towards strategic investment for health and wellbeing, focusing on outcomes, partnerships, independence and inclusion. It outlined eight steps for effective commissioning, including putting people at the centre of commissioning, understanding the needs of the population through the development of a JSNA and developing appropriate incentives. The latter could be channelled through local area agreements (LAAs) across a local authority area, contracts, pooled budgets, direct payments and through PBC. A WCC assessment framework was produced (Department of Health, 2007b), along with guidance and support, and an annual WCC assurance process was set in motion (Department of Health, 2008a, 2009a). The pressure on PCTs to achieve high levels of commissioning performance increased during the period of the study and was further prompted by the publication of a calibrated 'league table' of PCTs, combining scores for competencies and governance (Crump, 2009) and where performance was linked to the degree of commissioning autonomy granted to PCTs. It was intended to enable good practice to be identified through benchmarking across commissioning organisations but also rather undermined the original notion of WCC as a developmental process.

The study was completed just before the election of the coalition government in 2010, and the publication of the White Paper *Equity and excellence: Liberating the NHS* (Secretary of State for Health, 2010a), which signalled major changes in the governance arrangements of the NHS in England. These included the abolition of Strategic Health Authorities (SHAs) in 2012, of PCTs from 2013, the comprehensive area assessment (after one year of operation) in 2010, and arm's-length bodies, including the Health Protection Agency.

Fieldwork for the study therefore mirrored a period over which the WCC assurance framework shaped PCT commissioning activities, including commissioning for health and wellbeing. Some PCTs also made organisational changes, reconfiguring roles and responsibilities better to reflect their commissioning function. The following section describes the commissioning cycle and explores the ways in which commissioners interpreted the phrase 'commissioning for health and wellbeing', as this was likely to influence commissioning practice.

A public health-led approach to commissioning

The WCC programme was nothing if not ambitious, with the title itself inviting high expectations:

> So why use the phrase 'world class commissioning'? Put simply, it is a statement of intent, designed to raise ambitions for a new form of commissioning that has not yet been developed or implemented in a comprehensive way across

any of the developed healthcare economies. (Department of Health, 2007b: 1)

Although subsequently discarded, the WCC initiative nevertheless presented a clear and systematic approach to the principles of commissioning, set out the ordered phases of a continuous commissioning cycle, itemised competencies required for effective commissioning and established an annual assessment process. The influence of WCC as a performance management regime is further discussed in Chapter Four.

PCTs were assessed against three areas: governance, outcomes and competencies. Governance, in this case, referred to 'board grip', finance and whether the PCT board had taken ownership of a meaningful five-year strategic plan, supported by, and reflected in, a five-year financial plan. Ten health outcomes were assessed: two of the outcomes (improving life expectancy and addressing health inequalities) were mandatory and measured for all PCTs, with a further eight outcomes determined locally from a predetermined list of over 60 outcomes, chosen to be capable of measurement (so that progress could be monitored). Additional local targets could also be chosen by PCTs. There were 11 WCC competencies and each competency was associated with three key indicators (with each indicator assessed against a four-point scale). In addition, PCTs were also rated on a traffic light system for the three areas of governance. This made for a complicated assessment procedure.

For PCT interviewees in the study, WCC competencies were largely considered to have encouraged a systematic approach to the commissioning cycle, to knowledge management and to prioritisation. WCC had also meant that strategic and financial plans were developed in tandem and were closely aligned. It was argued that WCC was premised on a public health model:

> 'And I'm finding that doors that perhaps were a bit shut are starting to open because people are seeing the value of public health in world class commissioning terms. You can't just do cost and volume contracts any more. You've got to go down to the value and the efficiency and the effectiveness of your contracts, and that is public health. I mean you can't get away from the need for a public health analysis of these things even if you wanted to.' (DPH, site 1)

Box 3.1 lists the competencies and gives examples of indicators at the highest level of assessment (that is, level four) where these are relevant for promoting health and health equity. Relevant indicators included partnership working across the health and wellbeing agenda, proactive identification of populations at risk, meeting unmet needs of disadvantaged groups and investing for longer-term health gain. (The full list of indicators was included in a commissioning assurance handbook [Department of Health, 2009a]). While there were numerous indicators, taken together they provided a detailed account of what was expected of commissioners and how they could improve over time. Competencies were applied to a continuous commissioning cycle which involved assessing needs and services through the JSNA, identifying any gaps (or overprovision), prioritising investment in the light of available resources and then procuring services accordingly, which might involve 'stimulating' the market. Services would then be monitored and evaluated before the process began again. This process was often easier to apply to growth funding than to total spend or to disinvestment, however. Figure 3.1 illustrates the nature of the commissioning cycle at the time of the study.

Box 3.1: Commissioning competencies

1. Recognised as 'local leader' of the NHS, e.g. 'the PCT actively participates in and leads the local health agenda'.

2. Work collaboratively with community partners, e.g. 'there is clear clinical leadership... in creating, reconfirming and delivering the LAA'; 'multiple partnerships are in place across a broad range of settings to support and deliver the health and wellbeing agenda'.

3. Engage with the public and patients, e.g. 'key stakeholders strongly agree that the PCT proactively shapes health opinions and aspirations of the public and patients';'... proactive engagement and partnership arrangements with the local community... are embedded in all commissioning processes'.

4. Collaborate with clinicians.

5. Manage knowledge and assess needs, e.g. 'the PCT has proactive population risk stratification to identify populations at risk and to intervene at the earliest possible point';'the PCT has a view of unmet needs for disadvantaged sub-groups'; 'the PCT has developed plans to match the top performers on each benchmark'.

6. Prioritise investment of all spend, e.g.: 'predictive modelling to support its ability to target required interventions with precision'; 'understands the return on past investment (and disinvestment)'; 'mature programme budgeting... for all key priority care pathways/disease groups'; 'the PCT invests for longer-term health outcome gains and can quantify impact'.

7. Stimulate the market.

8. Promote improvement in quality through clinical and provider innovation.

9. Secure procurement skills, e.g. 'contract incentives drive desired provider performance which results in health improvements'.

10. Manage the local health system and work in partnership with providers.

11. Sound financial investments (this competency was originally assessed in the governance domain), e.g. 'the PCT improves efficiency and effectiveness of spend whilst delivering greater health benefits and improved quality'.

Figure 3.1: The commissioning cycle

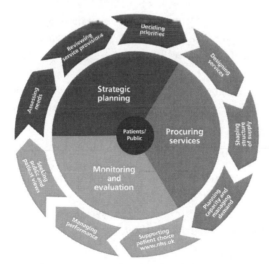

Source: Copyright © 2013, re-used with the permission of the Health and Social Care Information Centre. All rights reserved.

The starting point of a commissioning cycle is to assess the health needs of the population. Whether commissioning decisions result in improving population health and addressing inequalities depends on the quality of local health needs assessments and the extent to which these assessments influence priority setting and service development. Although the process of needs assessment plays a key role, it is also the case that implementation of each phase of the commissioning cycle may (or may not) serve to promote health improvement and the reduction of health inequalities. For example, equity considerations can be incorporated into the development of contracts, incentives and audit arrangements. While over half the sites considered that health and wellbeing was emphasised throughout the commissioning process, a preventive ethos in commissioning was also influenced by how NHS commissioners interpreted the phrase 'commissioning for health and wellbeing' and this topic is considered in the following section.

Interpreting commissioning for health and wellbeing

The study considered how commissioners understood 'commissioning for health and wellbeing' on the basis that this could influence how the commissioning cycle was implemented in practice and, in particular, the extent to which a preventive ethos was reflected. The *Commissioning framework for health and well-being* (Department of Health, 2007a: 10), which prefigured the WCC initiative, itself reflected different approaches to health and wellbeing, including:

- a shift towards services that are personal, sensitive to individual need and that maintain independence and dignity;
- a strategic reorientation towards promoting health and wellbeing, investing now to reduce future ill health costs;
- a stronger focus on commissioning the services and interventions that will achieve better health, across health and local government, with everyone working together to promote inclusion and tackle health inequalities.

The phrase was interpreted differently both within and across PCTs in the study. While the ambiguity of the term was noted, there were advantages in referring to both 'health' and 'wellbeing', as this helped to focus attention on the promotion of health rather than on the provision of health care:

> 'It keeps the preventative aspect on the agenda. You know, because it forces people to define health as opposed to health care. Because, you know, that's the danger if you're commissioning for health, then people will just think health services and then health care, whereas health and wellbeing reminds them that it's much more than that.' (DPH, site 2)

However, health needed to be distinguished from wellbeing: one interviewee noted, for example, that the social gradient for health was not the same as the social gradient for wellbeing:

> 'But there are some important findings that come out, not least the different distribution of health and wellbeing and they're commonly put together in a common phrase with almost the implication that if you improve health you improve wellbeing and vice versa. It's very clear that things like the social class gradient for health are not the same as the social class gradient for wellbeing.... I'm confident with the drivers of health and I know what we need to do to tackle those. I'm not so sure we have a clear understanding of what the real drivers of wellbeing are.' (PCT chief executive, site 3)

Four main aspects of 'commissioning for health and wellbeing' were in evidence across interviewees in the study.

Public health values are mainstreamed

> 'All the commissioning plans start in the public health directorate.' (Director of strategy, site 3)

> 'I want public health values to pervade the entire organisation. I want basically commissioning to think in public health terms for when they commission rather than in health management terms.' (DPH, site 1)

As illustrated in the above quotations, in this approach, the aspiration was for public health to be fully mainstreamed in the commissioning cycle and for public health values to pervade decision-making processes and not be seen as the sole preserve of a public health department or of public health professionals. The same DPH commented:

'The worst thing in the world is to see commissioning for health and wellbeing as being primarily a public health role. That's the worst thing in the world; it's got to be the bread and butter of commissioning, mainstream commissioning.' (DPH, site 1)

In some PCTs in the study, roles and responsibilities were being restructured and remodelled to reflect a 'public health organisation', for example, through the merger of strategic and public health directorates, to reflect the key public health role in strategic commissioning. In these cases, commissioning for health and wellbeing was seen as synonymous with the role of a commissioning organisation, with the whole of the commissioning cycle, 'the total business of this organisation'. For example, one DPH described it as follows:

'Right, well, it would mean identifying the health needs, identifying appropriate interventions, service specifications and then either testing the market or asking existing providers to deliver a set of standards, monitoring it and evaluating it.' (DPH, site 4)

In two sites, public health was described as at the heart of this process:

'We don't have a directorate of commissioning ... commissioning's what the organisation does, not what a directorate does ... we've broken commissioning down into its component parts.... And when we looked at what strategy and planning was all about in terms of that part of the commissioning cycle ... well that's what public health teams do.' (Director of strategy, site 3)

However, this integrated approach was not widespread and over half the PCTs in the study included interviewees who considered that 'silo working' in public health teams had created a barrier to commissioning for health and wellbeing. Moreover, it was argued that directorates had different priorities and separate skills would be required for each phase of the commissioning cycle. Not all interviewees were enthusiastic about a split between commissioning and providing public health services in the first place. It was argued, for example, that public health staff often performed both a commissioner and a provider role, and that being integrated into all aspects of the commissioning cycle could distract public health teams away from their advocacy role in promoting a public health perspective. Nevertheless, there was generally little direct provision of public health services. For example, healthy lifestyle interventions were often commissioned through health trainers, the voluntary and community sector (VCS), community pharmacists and general practice.

Commissioning through partnerships

Interviewees were clear that commissioning for health and wellbeing mainly involved focusing 'upstream', addressing social determinants of health and working across local partnerships in close collaboration with local authorities. Some interviewees considered tackling inequalities between different localities or wards as a key priority, while others focused more specifically on partnerships across agencies to address lifestyle risk factors and interventions related to smoking cessation, reducing obesity or promoting exercise. There were examples of shared health and wellbeing funds across PCTs and local authorities, joint posts for developing local neighbourhood approaches and joint approaches to employing health trainers. In commissioning for health and wellbeing, it was considered important to consider effects across the whole health economy. However, financial stringency could threaten these partnership initiatives. A narrowing of the preventive agenda was described by one DPH as follows:

> 'I think what's happened in the last year, in particular, and the current financial forecast for the NHS has made us very much refocus on NHS services again, and in a way it's to the detriment of some of the partnership agendas that we were exploring through our public health roles in the organisation ... now it's a very tight NHS focus and getting much more efficiencies out of the NHS, and it may well be to the detriment of broader public health programmes I think.' (DPH, site 6)

Commissioning public health services

Reflecting a narrower view of the role of public health professionals in commissioning, this approach focused on commissioning services for secondary prevention and lifestyle interventions, partly as a reaction to limited public health resources.

> 'I think yes, you could look at it both ways. I mean you could look at it and say well actually why is public health not being more actively engaged in core mainstream commissioning, or you could say actually there's a limited public health resource and where do we want to put the emphasis ... a fundamental part of our role is to get resources out of traditional commissioning and into lifestyle services. And so to some extent I think we have a role there in terms of questioning it but I don't think that means that we need to sit on each commissioning group.' (DPH, site 8 in Marks et al., 2011c: 16)

Commissioning for health and wellbeing as NHS business

In this approach, the one most commonly adopted, commissioning for health and wellbeing was seen as the sum of existing NHS activities, the 'total business' of the organisation, spanning prevention, care and rehabilitation across a pathway of care, as each commissioning decision was ultimately related to the health and wellbeing of patients and this could be improved across all stages of a pathway of care. It was particularly the case that practice-based commissioners focused on pathway redesign and on the relocation of services from secondary to primary care:

> 'I mean, well, commissioning isn't that old anyway and therefore in the first couple of years of commissioning, you've got to go for the big hits really and prescribing and scheduled care alternatives to hospital for kind of outpatient type procedures and surgery, these are all the obvious early areas of work. I think once you've got beyond that bulge, which has to happen first I think, then we certainly as a cluster have started to think on the health and wellbeing strategy.' (PBC lead, site 2)

> 'They've actually gone in and looked at their full pathway of care and really redesigned the way patients flow through the system to improve the patient experience, which again in itself does improve the health and wellbeing.' (Director of finance, site 6)

Others focused on long-term conditions and improved access to primary care.

'And so we want to do two things. We want to focus initially on helping people to manage themselves with long-term conditions. What we then want to do is move down the triangle to prevent things happening.' (PCT operating director, site 8)

A public health approach to care pathway development would inject a population perspective throughout, shifting the focus of commissioning decisions away from 'decision trees for treatment' towards preventive services.

Commissioning for health and wellbeing could, therefore, be pursued through a public health-led approach across the whole care pathway or could simply describe the status quo, in that it redefined all NHS activity as commissioning for health and wellbeing. The latter view was reflected in over half the sites and showed that ambiguity associated with the term had its dangers. If everything was redefined as health and wellbeing, there was risk that a focus on prevention would be lost, especially given financial pressures. The extent to which commissioning organisations reflect a public health ethos and invest in health over the longer-term is likely to come under increasing threat in a context of reduced public spending.

Joint strategic needs assessments

While the extent to which a public health ethos was reflected throughout the commissioning cycle varied across sites, health needs assessment remains the starting point for a public health-led approach to commissioning. It provides a basis for priority setting, service development or reconfiguration and for addressing inequalities in access to services. In particular, it can help to avoid the dangers of reproducing historic patterns of provision which may not reflect changes in demography, morbidity, technology or treatment. JSNAs have the potential to question the status quo in the interests of population health but only if they act as a lever for subsequent commissioning decisions and are reflected in decisions made throughout the commissioning cycle.

The starting point of a JSNA is an analysis of current health and social care needs (as well as of projected future needs) rather than of the demand for health or social care, which may not fully reflect need. JSNAs can include analysis of health inequalities between different groups and areas, local social and environmental factors influencing health, and the needs of disadvantaged, underserved or socially excluded groups. They can be informed by health equity audits demonstrating any gaps between the need for services and their distribution and, over time, can help to assess the impact of investments, policies and services on health and health inequalities. Box 3.2 lists information included in JSNAs.

Box 3.2: Building the joint strategic needs assessment

Although there is no formal template, JSNAs can include the following data drawing on national datasets, local health profiles, indices of deprivation and neighbourhood statistics:

- demographic data (total population, growth, migration, birth rates, gender, age composition, ethnicity);
- social and place-related data (housing quality, environment, green space, employment, educational attainment, benefit uptake, crime and disorder and community cohesion);
- lifestyle determinants (exercise, smoking, diet, alcohol, drug abuse);
- morbidity and mortality data (life expectancy, incidence and prevalence of ill health, including non-communicable diseases); projections over time; immunisation uptake rates; long-standing illness; use of social care services;
- service access and utilisation, including uptake of preventive services; assessments of reported against expected prevalence; access to services in disadvantaged areas or for vulnerable groups; benchmarked data on spend and outcomes; value for money;
- community views (expectations, perceptions and experiences of service users and local communities about what contributes to good health). A range of methods should be available to gather community perspectives, including surveys, complaints and scrutiny reports;
- projections of health status and of service use.

These data sources can be supplemented with further information, reflecting the nature of the local community, although baseline information related to inequalities in health and access to health care (by locality, by socio-economic group and for black and minority ethnic groups) may not be routinely available. From an equity focus, for example, the JSNA should include:

- inequalities (by geographical area, socioeconomic status, ethnicity, gender);
- inequalities in risk factors, prevalence of diseases, life expectancy;
- life expectancy gaps between wards, boroughs and compared with the national average;
- services needed compared with services available;
- inequity of access to primary care and health care services;

- distribution of expenditure in relation to need;
- locality-based analyses.

Since 2008, there has been a plethora of advice, good practice examples and guidance related to health profiles and JSNAs, in order to promote a population-based approach to needs assessment and an emphasis on health outcomes rather than on services, processes and outputs. Minimum data sets for JSNAs were established (including a core data set with the original guidance [Department of Health, 2007d]), developed through the Association of Public Health Observatories and the Local Government Association (Brotherton and Battersby, 2011) and *A springboard for action* (Harding et al., 2011) (which provided a toolkit with issues for debate in each of the key areas of the JSNA), the NHS Confederation (NHS Confederation, 2011a) and further guidance (Department of Health, 2013a). Identification of unmet needs could also be derived from the VCS and local Healthwatch. Separate annual health profiles for each local authority area (which had been produced by Public Health Observatories from 2006) provided a snapshot of health for each local authority in England and useful comparative information (including a 'spine chart' health summary showing the differences between the area and the average for England for 32 health-related indicators). Together with evidence of the cost-effectiveness of interventions, these provide information to help commissioners plan and prioritise services.

Nationally, there are examples of excellence in building on JSNAs in developing commissioning priorities. For example, the former NHS Tower Hamlets developed an award-winning strategy, informed by local health needs assessments, to identify priorities across the borough, with key actions determined through multi-agency events and public forums. Key priorities included improving primary care and actively addressing under-diagnosis; the development of social marketing techniques; using community intelligence; and targeting areas of greatest need.

Although the statutory requirement for producing a JSNA for each local authority area dates from 2008, there is a long tradition of carrying out assessments of the health of local populations, originating in annual reports of Medical Officers of Health (MOsH), which started in 1847 and continued until the post of the MOH came to an end in 1972 (swiftly followed by the reorganisation of the NHS in 1974, which moved public health out of local government). Health care needs assessments for specific topics have been carried out since the 1990s (Marshall and Hothersall, 2012) and follow a logical procedure (rapid assessment; analysis of need; [cost]-effective interventions; current service provision; matching supply to need; and implementation).[2]

Independent annual reports of DsPH, a requirement since 1988, also provide an analysis of local health needs and recommendations for improving population health.

In practice, there is often a mismatch between public health needs and the configuration of health care services and, as discussed in Chapter Six, there are many other influences on priority setting. At the time of the study, for example, these included the agenda for improving services set out in Lord Darzi's report, *High quality health care for all* (Secretary of State for Health, 2008), published just before the first-phase interviews, where local commissioning strategies were required to reflect its recommendations. However, the introduction of JSNAs signalled an important shift in emphasis.

First of all, a JSNA for a local population was placed on a statutory basis. The Local Government and Public Involvement in Health Act 2007 (section 116) required PCTs and upper-tier local authorities to produce, from 2008, a JSNA of the health and wellbeing of their local community. This was to be achieved through collaboration across DsPH, adult social services and children's services. The requirement to carry out a JSNA had been prefigured in the White Papers, *Our health, our care, our say* (Secretary of State for Health, 2006) and *Strong and prosperous communities* (Secretary of State for Communities and Local Government, 2006).

Second, the JSNA was originally intended as a joint endeavour across PCTs and local authorities to encourage partnership working. The Local Government and Public Involvement in Health Act placed a new duty to cooperate on PCTs and local authorities, working together on JSNAs, identifying the health needs of the local population and aligning it with other strategic plans, such as the Children and Young People's Plans and housing strategies of the local authority. In the same vein, the *Commissioning framework for health and well-being* (Department of Health, 2007a), noted that:

> Local leaders and decision-makers need to develop an improved shared understanding of the health and social care needs of their local population, a joint vision and an integrated approach to improving health and wellbeing, reducing inequalities and promoting health equity. (para. 15)

A wide range of stakeholders was originally envisaged, although in practice this proved difficult to achieve. However, the JSNA was designed to promote strategic planning across partners, including voluntary organisations and the private sector through a shared understanding of needs and priorities.

Third, JSNAs were the first step in the commissioning cycle and designed to be integrated with it, informing and influencing commissioning priorities, market development and investment decisions. Through the WCC initiative, progress of PCTs in jointly developing JSNAs and the extent to which the JSNA informed the commissioning cycle was performance managed through the Department of Health. For example, of the 10 targets for improved health outcomes, eight could be chosen locally (given certain restrictions) and these could be derived from the JSNA. Guidance (Department of Health, 2007d: 6) stated that:

> The WCC competencies emphasise the role of JSNA in driving the long term commissioning strategies of PCTs and their collaborative work with community partners, and include an emphasis on public and patient engagement.

There was therefore a clear route through which the JSNA could make a difference to commissioning decisions. This remained the case post-2010, where *Equity and excellence* (Secretary of State for Health, 2010a) maintained the central role of the JSNA, to be led by local authorities in collaboration with others (under the duty of partnership) through statutory health and wellbeing boards (HWBs). JSNAs would be reflected in new joint health and wellbeing strategies and were intended to influence decisions on investment and disinvestment. Subsequent guidance (Department of Health, 2013a: 4) reiterated that:

> Their outputs, in the form of evidence and the analysis of needs, and agreed priorities, will be used to help to determine what actions local authorities, the local NHS and other partners need to take to meet health and social care needs, and to address the wider determinants that impact on health and wellbeing.

Fourth, was an emphasis on incorporating views of local communities, including seldom heard and vulnerable groups and not just those of existing users of services or health and social care professionals. Although there was variation in the extent to which this was achieved, some PCTs, jointly with local authorities, developed innovative methods for analysing and addressing inequalities in their local populations, engaging the views of local communities, including groups whose views were often overlooked. It was also an opportunity for local communities to become involved in identifying local priorities for investment or disinvestment:

> A good strategic needs assessment ... is based on a joint analysis of current and predicted health and wellbeing outcomes, an account of what people in the local community want from their services (those provided by the statutory sector and the wider market), and a view of the future, predicting and anticipating potential new or unmet need. It could include opportunities for disinvestment and resource transfer. And it should incorporate views of the local population, not just existing users of services, and include and be informed by equality impact assessments. (Department of Health, 2007a: para. 3.10)

It was noted that this was the biggest challenge for JSNAs and that the NHS needed to build on the experience of local authorities in engaging with their local communities. This theme is continued in later guidance (Department of Health 2013a) with the additional emphasis on 'supporting active communities' and building on community assets. Local Healthwatch is intended to engage with local communities in relation to their experience of health and social care services.

Fifth, was a future orientation, anticipating future needs as well as current demand and unmet need as a spur to commissioning for longer-term outcomes. The relevance to future need was also emphasised in the Health and Social Care Act 2012. Predictive modelling techniques and scenario planning, sometimes in conjunction with local authorities, were developed by some PCTs in the study. However, as further discussed in Chapter Six, while prioritising allocation for a whole population involves matching services to needs for particular problems, it also raises broader ethical, resource and political issues where the JSNA forms only one influence on decision making.

JSNAs were continued as a statutory requirement by the coalition government under the Health and Social Care Act 2012, but amended to refer to local authority HWBs. Post-April 2013, local authorities and CCGs have 'equal and joint duties' to prepare JSNAs and joint health and wellbeing strategies, led by HWBs (section 193 of the Act) which are established by each upper-tier local authority (section 194). The Act (section 192) clarifies that CCGs that share boundaries with a local authority have a duty to prepare a JSNA, and that the local authority has a duty to publish a Joint Health and Wellbeing Strategy.

CCGs, local authorities and NHS England all have to take account of needs and priorities identified in the JSNA, while CCG plans should be consistent with JSNAs and any inconsistencies justified. HWBs have the right to challenge these plans if they depart from JSNAs – and can, if necessary, appeal to NHS England and the Secretary of State for Health, although it is unclear whether this will happen in practice. Public concern related to local authority responses to the JSNA and joint health and wellbeing strategies can be addressed through council leaders and scrutiny committees as part of the democratic process. The requirement for CCG involvement is, perhaps, an attempt to rectify the relatively limited involvement of GPs (through PBC) in developing the JSNA during the period of WCC.

Statutory guidance on the JSNA and joint health and wellbeing strategies (Department of Health, 2013a) reflects a version of the WCC cycle for HWBs, emphasising the key role of the JSNA and the importance of transparency and accountability in the process (see Figure 3.2), although there is less emphasis on health inequalities, neighbourhoods, poverty and environmental aspects, which had figured prominently in the guidance for JSNAs introduced in the *Commissioning framework for health and well-being* (Department of Health, 2007a).

Much is expected of JSNAs. The study explored the views of interviewees in 2008–9, when JSNAs were still at a relatively early stage:

Figure 3.2: JSNA and joint health and wellbeing strategies

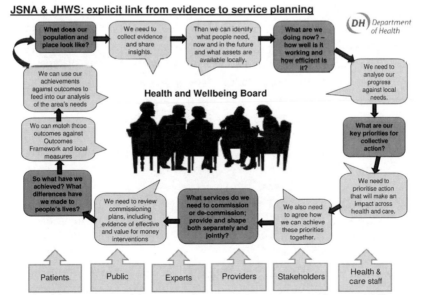

Source: Department of Health (2013a) Licensed under the Open Government Licence

the first round of JSNAs had just been completed when interviews began. However, they provide an indication of progress and potential tensions. The following areas are explored: variation in developing the JSNA and in the impact of the JSNA on the commissioning cycle; the extent to which it reflected partnership working; and the involvement of GPs through PBC. Involvement of the VCS and of local authority scrutiny committees in the JSNA was also explored and is discussed in more detail in Chapter Seven.

Local views of joint strategic needs assessments

There were different views over the usefulness of the JSNA. For some interviewees, it was considered a formalisation of what was already known and therefore added nothing new to commissioning intentions. It was argued that population needs did not vary greatly from year to year and data were already available through the annual DPH report. For the majority, however, the JSNA was perceived as a spur to wider partnership working, formalising disparate processes and providing a firm basis for commissioning. Some interviewees questioned the extent to which expectations for the JSNA had been fulfilled in practice, namely whether JSNAs were built on joint approaches to assessing needs, whether they encouraged data sharing or triangulation of data, and whether they had influenced priority setting in both the PCT and the local authority. It was argued that the JSNA should be a constantly developing evidence-based resource across the different partners, rather than a 'glossy document'. For example, a core database could be made available online, jointly shared and linked to more detailed health needs assessments. Interviewees were positive about the potential of joint commissioning approaches for improving preventive services. A director of strategy noted:

> 'My feeling is no, actually that is something we really should be commissioning together because then we can make the synergies with library services, leisure services, in a much more joined up way than we are just by commissioning children to go and see a dietician or whatever. We could do some really clever stuff if we had that joint ownership of the problem between the two of us.' (Site 3)

There was wide variation in JSNAs in the study: some were brief or largely descriptive while others made commissioning recommendations, identified local targets and made links with commissioning processes in the local authority. Some were combined with the independent annual report of the DPH, while in other cases the DPH report provided a more detailed account of health needs and priorities for service development than did the JSNA. There was also great variation in data availability and in the existence of data resources shared across PCTs and local authorities. While public health teams and local authority managers from the relevant directorates were routinely involved in developing JSNAs, progress was influenced by the extent to which there was already a shared data platform: two sites had jointly funded data observatories, for example, and a number of others had long-standing joint arrangements for collating and presenting findings. Geographical focus (city, county, borough) also varied. JSNAs refer to a local authority area and could therefore relate to a number of PCTs or a number of district councils.

Perhaps of greater significance was the extent to which area profiles or a locality focus were included in the JSNA, and whether detailed locality profiles were linked to locality commissioning and to programmes directly targeted to meet the needs of local communities. In four sites, the JSNA was locality based or was being developed in this direction. In one of these sites, for example, the JSNA had brought together a wide range of information around local communities with a number of area profiles supported by smaller locality profiles. It was informed by widespread canvassing of views and feedback from local communities, the VCS and PBC, and tied into locality commissioning arrangements with PBC. This exercise had demonstrated variation across a wide range of sectors, ranging from education to the availability of, and access to, health services. It had also served to highlight variations in access to services between localities, to identify 'priority communities' and had helped to align priorities across local organisations, such as district councils, PCTs and county councils.

This had resulted in some priority communities being identified in order better to target resources. Ironically, these initiatives often referred back to primary care groups, which had pre-dated PCTs, but had achieved a greater locality focus and were described by a director of strategic commissioning (site 10), for example, as having 'more local empowerment, responsibility and accountability'.

There was variation in the extent to which the JSNA was considered a joint document with the local authority, reflected, for example, in the existence of JSNA leads in the local authority, an evidence base shared across the PCT and local authority, alignment with key themes of local authority sustainable community strategies and a shared definition of key concepts, such as needs assessment. It was noted by some PCT interviewees that local authorities often considered PCTs responsible for health: health needs assessments could conjure up quite different tasks in the two organisations, often associated in the local authority with responding to public demands. In two of the ten case study sites, the JSNA had been led by the local authority and, in one site, there had been difficulties over sharing health and local authority data. There were examples of joint working, however, and of taking joint approaches from the outset. For example, one site chose a purposive approach, focusing on areas where not enough information was available, there were joint concerns and action could be taken on findings.

> 'So for each of those projects there's someone from the public health department, there's a local authority officer and there's a steering group above it. So every project has ... local authority/public health working together on an area of joint concern.' (Associate DPH, site 5)

Another site chose to triangulate information from different sources to test assumptions and used scenario modelling techniques to indicate future service needs.

Having just completed the first round of JSNAs at the time of first-phase interviews, PCTs viewed them as work in progress. Interviewees in a majority of sites claimed that the JSNA had improved links between health and social care, made the use of information more systematic and, in some cases, had informed the work of joint health and social care teams, promoting a shared understanding of concepts and helping to develop joint commissioning. One DPH commented:

> 'So I suppose the difference the joint strategic needs assessment has made is it is a more systematic approach to looking at data sources and making judgements, drawing hypotheses about what those data sources tell you in a way that we haven't been able to do before. So that's really helpful, and because our services are joined up, we have joint health and social care teams, that makes a lot of sense in planning terms.' (Site 10)

In one site, there had been extensive public involvement with over 3,000 responses gained through a large consultative exercise, leaflet drops and a media campaign, and in another there had been numerous stakeholder events and the public was also involved in a strategic commissioning forum and in discussions over priority setting. However, as discussed in Chapter Seven, local authority Overview and Security Committees (OSCs) were largely unaware of the JSNA and local involvement networks had been involved in one site only.

Overall, there was recognition in the study that the JSNA should help influence commissioning decisions and priorities, develop locality planning, target interventions and services, and promote links between health and social care. However, there was variation in length, quality and relevance, and whether a locality focus was adopted. There were differences in the history of collaboration, including over data sharing, and these affected its effectiveness. As the first stage in the commissioning cycle, JSNAs needed to be reflected in decision making and priority setting if they were to be other than a 'tick box' exercise.

Addressing health inequalities through commissioning

While they have the potential to highlight inequalities and inform commissioning decisions JSNAs also run the risk of being poorly integrated into the rest of the commissioning cycle. In order to address the social gradient in health, commissioners need to build on the information in JSNAs to target services and work across relevant partnerships. The following section looks at ways in which commissioners can address local inequalities in health and considers barriers and enablers identified in the study.

Local interventions

Commissioners can try to address inequalities in a number of different ways, including action on the social determinants of health; improving access to primary care services; systematically addressing contributors to the life expectancy gap (for which interactive tools have been developed); addressing under-diagnosis (through comparing expected with reported prevalence); using community intelligence; and targeting groups and areas of disadvantage. Advice on 'high impact' changes to reduce health inequalities was made available to commissioners, including a health inequalities intervention tool (see Chapter Six). While some interventions involve commissioning specific services, addressing social determinants of health at a local level requires partnership working to align policies and priorities. Action on six policy objectives identified by Marmot's review of health inequalities in England, *Fair society, healthy lives* (Marmot Review, 2010), is intended to address the social gradient in health across the life course, and is particularly relevant for local authorities:

- give every child the best start in life;
- enable all children, young people and adults to maximise their capabilities and have control over their lives;
- create fair employment and good work for all;
- ensure a healthy standard of living for all;
- create and develop healthy and sustainable places and communities;
- strengthen the role and impact of ill health prevention.

How services are targeted is also important. The phrase 'proportionate universalism' has been used to reflect the fact that 'actions must be universal, but with a scale and intensity that is proportionate to the level of disadvantage' (Marmot Review, 2010: 16). Otherwise, improving population health overall may be accompanied by a widening of health inequalities.

Many targeted initiatives to improve health and address inequalities were being implemented by PCTs and local authorities at the time of the study, not least given the requirements of national health inequalities targets, mandatory health outcomes for WCC and a wide range of other relevant targets (further described in Chapter Four). In addition, PCTs had established their own local targets in areas such as smoking cessation and addressing premature mortality, often focused on disadvantaged groups and areas. For the life expectancy targets, as discussed elsewhere, there was often an emphasis on clinical preventive interventions as a route for meeting the national health inequalities targets (Blackman et al., 2006), focusing on controlling cardiovascular disease through treating hypertension, reducing cholesterol levels and through smoking cessation services. Clarity about the timescales involved was essential, however, as one interviewee commented:

> '[The] PCT has got to be transparent about what its time horizons are. Because if you say all right, it's only about five years, then around healthy lifestyles you might as well decommission all the children's stuff and to an extent adult obesity services because the only thing that will really have an impact if you're looking this very very narrow way is smoking cessation, you know, if that's the logic you want to follow. But then if the PCT are saying well actually we do have an investment in the future health of children and the things that we are investing in currently will only have an impact in 10 to 20 years, then it has to say that.' (Assistant DPH, site 5)

Box 3.3 summarises approaches adopted by PCTs and local authorities for reducing premature mortality in disadvantaged groups and areas (focusing on initiatives for smoking cessation and statin prescription) at the time the study began, in 2007, and based on a separate mapping exercise (see Marks et al., 2007, for further discussion). These were limited to specific interventions shown to reduce premature mortality rather than upstream interventions, but the approaches in Box 3.3 were often used in combination and as part of wider health promotion initiatives. Equity audits, combined with knowledge of local communities and a flexible, user friendly approach were important routes for targeting local inequalities. Services needed to be accessible and convenient but also relevant for the groups in question. A range of incentive schemes for meeting preventive targets was deployed through the general medical services (GMS) and pharmacy contracts (and these are discussed in the context of the study in Chapter Five). Despite the priority attached to addressing inequalities over this period, many services specifically targeted at disadvantaged groups or areas were set up as pilots, with short-term funding, typically in response to additional funding being made available, rather than through changes in mainstream budgets. This made them vulnerable when NHS growth funds dried up. In the new arrangements, public health support is to be provided to CCGs to help meet the needs of vulnerable groups, and this can include geo-demographic profiling to help identify a mismatch between need for services and utilisation for target groups.

Box 3.3: Identifying and reaching underserved groups
1. Identifying target populations

* ward-based approaches: identifying deprivation by ward/super output area using the Index of Multiple Deprivation (IMD) and estimating prevalence;
* proactive case finding of high-risk patients through GP practice registers (may focus on practices in disadvantaged areas or population-based screening);
* equity audits (used to identify under-diagnosis, inequalities in service planning and delivery and measure effectiveness over time);
* lifestyle surveys (using Health Survey for England, Household Panel Survey or carrying out local surveys);
* client databases;
* local mapping exercises;
* geo-demographic tools such as Mosaic: this is a geo-demographic tool that classifies all UK consumers into 11 distinct lifestyle groups and, within those groups, 61 types based on socioeconomic and sociocultural behaviour;

- comparing observed prevalence from GP practices (for example, from Quality and Outcomes Framework (QOF) data on smoking and statin prescription) with expected prevalence.

2. Reaching target groups

- using results from health equity audits to target activities;
- contacting smokers (by letter or through telemarketing) identified from GP practice/disease registers. GPs are already incentivised to record smoking prevalence;
- providing additional support to GP practices, especially practices in disadvantaged areas;
- targeting particular wards/neighbourhoods/estates/rural areas/Sure Start areas through a range of approaches;
- providing incentives through the local enhanced services element of GMS and pharmacy contracts; incentivising improved performance against QOF indicators;
- providing interpreting services;
- opportunistic screening (roadshows, mobile services, workplaces, targeting services in disadvantaged wards; sporadic initiatives [for example, Health MOTs in community locations]);
- proactive case finding through pharmacies: exploiting high street locations, long opening hours and marketing skills;
- community-based proactive approaches (one-stop shops, roving clinics);
- targeting specific groups (for example, pregnant women in disadvantaged areas and including home visits; black and minority ethnic groups in areas of high social deprivation).

3. Providing user friendly services

- culture-sensitive and responsive services: flexible drop-in services; rolling programmes for smoking cessation; community-based accessible services (pubs, clubs, leisure centres, job centres); stop smoking shops; pharmacies providing smoking cessation support and health checks; portable booths/ health buses;
- combined approaches (healthy lifestyle/keep fit initiatives) through community projects and social enterprises and delivered through a variety of settings;
- social marketing techniques to tailor health messages to specific (or 'segmented') groups. Social marketing is premised on understanding motivations of different groups and communities and tailoring services accordingly;
- lay health advisors: this includes outreach workers, peer educators and advocates; health trainers for lifestyle support;
- health checks in community settings/community-based clinics;
- financial and other incentives for lifestyle change.

In the study, the VCS was considered key for helping to address health inequalities and in one site, for example, all the smoking cessation services had been commissioned from a VCS provider. It was argued that the VCS could provide detailed knowledge and understanding of local communities, and had the ability to respond quickly. As discussed in Chapter Seven, the emphasis on competitive tendering can work against smaller VCS organisations, even though these organisations are most likely to be able to capitalise on local community engagement. Interviewees expressed concerns over the ability of the smaller VCS organisations to survive the move from receiving grants to competing in an open market and questioned whether they had the skills required to prepare tenders. At the time of the study, PCTs were assisting VCS organisations to develop the skills required for a market environment (as had been suggested in the *Commissioning framework for health and well-being* [Department of Health, 2007a: 39]). However, smaller VCS organisations were perceived as at risk.

With the transfer of public health into local authorities there is a broader scope for action, working across local authority directorates, carrying out health inequality impact assessments across policies and building on the strengths of local communities (Local Government Association, 2014).

Enablers and barriers

In order to support PCTs in the fifth most disadvantaged areas in England (designated as 'Spearhead' areas), the Health Inequalities National Support Team (one of several Department of Health national support teams) carried out on-site analyses at the time of the study. They shared good practice and subsequently summarised the knowledge they had distilled through their extensive programme of visits. This development approach assisted PCTs in meeting the national health inequalities targets. The National Support Team emphasised 'ten major lessons learned to date' (Bentley, 2008: 4–5) for addressing health inequalities locally, summarised below:

- make vision and strategy clear – taking a strategic and evidence-based approach including short-, medium- and longer-term strategies;
- extend leadership and engagement – lead from the top;
- make partnership work – this includes partnerships at all levels and the contribution of voluntary, community and faith organisations should be supported;

- get system and scale right – effective population-level interventions, addressing 'ad hoc and patchy delivery';
- adjust workforce – to suit 'industrial-scale' programmes;
- strengthen primary care in disadvantaged areas, challenge practices causing concern and support proactive primary care;
- find the 'missing thousands' – proactively identify those who are ill or at high risk who are not seeking care, using practice records and community outreach;
- capitalise on community engagement, especially those 'seldom seen and seldom heard';
- 'raise the bar' on target achievement in order to incentivise meeting the needs of those not accessing services and ensure that the vulnerable are not excluded from target registers;
- utilise population health intelligence and ensure adequate public health data and intelligence are available in real time. Analytical output should be disseminated and 'marketed' widely to stakeholders.

Many of these initiatives, as well as broader lessons for addressing inequalities, were reflected in the study. As Figure 3.3 demonstrates, the national survey showed that leadership and board commitment were the most important factors for enabling the health and wellbeing agenda.

Figure 3.3: Enablers for commissioning for health and wellbeing

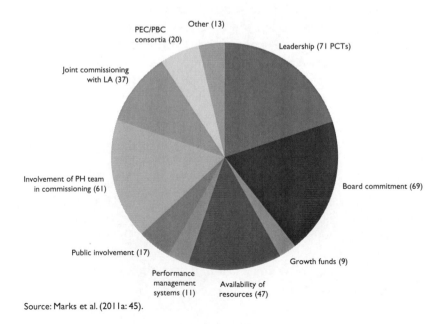

Source: Marks et al. (2011a: 45).

The PCT board played a key role in influencing values which informed criteria used in prioritisation processes. In six of the case study sites, leadership of the chief executive and the DPH was considered key to ensuring that public health priorities were reflected throughout the commissioning cycle. One participant noted:

> 'Our non-executive directors on the board are very much focused on the whole health inequalities agenda and, again, as part of that board they're a very crucial part of ensuring that we keep on that line and, you know, there is no doubt the whole health inequalities agenda is now running through the organisation like the words on a bit of rock.' (Director of finance, site 9 in Marks et al., 2011c: 17)

These findings were also reflected in focus group discussions and interviewee accounts. In one site, addressing weaknesses in primary care had been a priority and all sites had developed incentive schemes to encourage preventive activity in primary care (see Chapter Five). The importance of public health leaders telling 'a compelling story' was key in galvanising support among board members and others. Public involvement in commissioning was less developed, however.

Involvement of PBC in commissioning

Of particular relevance, given the role of CCGs in commissioning and their involvement in HWBs and joint health and wellbeing strategies, is the role of PBC in commissioning for health and wellbeing at the time of the study. *The commissioning framework for health and wellbeing* (Department of Health, 2007a: 8) described the JSNA as a joint endeavour across councils, PCTs and practice-based commissioners. It noted that 'GP practices will not only want to shape the JSNA but deliver the outcomes on a day to day basis' (2007a: 68). This is not dissimilar to current expectations of CCGs, although expectations that CCGs will engage have been made more explicit. In practice, GP involvement was limited and the JSNA was not used to develop commissioning priorities. In first-phase interviews, only one PBC lead had been involved in the JSNA process. While business cases for service development prepared by practice-based commissioners had to demonstrate relevance to the JSNA, interview data demonstrated little involvement with (as opposed to knowledge of) the JSNA. This reflects the wider issue of the often tangential relationship between PBC and PCT commissioning processes. The minimal involvement of

GPs in the JSNA was consistent with their lack of involvement in the commissioning cycle as a whole, although there was some variation across sites. However, it was important to engage general practices in addressing the health of their practice populations:

> 'There isn't something that takes place in the community and something separate that takes place in the surgery, they're the same population so we really ought to get better at joining the dots up, so there's a way to go there.' (Director of strategy, site 7)

There were often poor working relationships across small PBC groups and between these commissioning groups and the PCT. Interviewees attributed the lack of involvement in commissioning to a number of reasons, not least of which was a lack of capacity on the part of clinicians to take on these extra tasks, and, in practice, PBC was dependent on a relatively small number of enthusiasts. Roles were still being developed and tensions arose from the bureaucratic burden involved in commissioning and conflicts of interest as GPs were both providers and commissioners. There were also clear tensions for PBC interviewees between what was perceived as central control by PCTs and their need for local autonomy.

However, a few PCT interviewees described active commissioning consortia leading the response to strategic plans, and acting as a driving force. They were also able to translate 'policy ideas into something that works locally'. As one interviewee put it:

> 'And therefore practice-based commissioning, if used properly, harnesses the intellect, knowledge, experience and understanding of the local population to the corporate strategy of the organisation, uses their performance management reporting, i.e. they get on a daily basis the outcomes and experience patients have of the system, to shape, inform and influence the PCT planning processes.' (Director of strategy, site 2)

Although demand management had always figured prominently in PBC, second-phase interviews reflected an increased emphasis on this area, often centrally driven and reinforced through tighter targets for elective care. The focus was, therefore, on clinical forums, service redesign, providing care closer to home, and developing pathways of care. This might involve working across larger population groups in order to develop the critical mass needed to inform commissioning decisions, particularly in relation to secondary care. In some case study sites, pathway redesign was in its early stages, focused on areas such as physiotherapy and dermatology.

Practice-based commissioners were viewed as innovators or as providing communication channels between general practices and the PCT. In one site, some PBC consortia were involved with local health and wellbeing partnerships, and in another the PCT was working with practice-based commissioners in locality-based commissioning, as reflected in the JSNA. Some interviewees highlighted benefits of greater involvement and one interviewee commented on the benefits of involving GPs with the JSNA process in particular, as it helped demonstrate how their activities fitted into city-wide benefits. In the majority of sites, links were being developed between public health teams and PBC consortia: public health support included analysis of public health data for PBC clusters, membership of PBC boards or involvement with PBC leads. Information for consortia could include relative performance on hospital admissions or comparative data on premature mortality rates, although there were sometimes problems in reconciling ward and practice population data. Or PBC consortia could be provided with a menu of preventive interventions, as in the example, below:

> 'So [DPH] kind of gave us a sheet and said these are the kind of initiatives that we'd like you to do. It was up to PBC then in a variety of ways to look across their population and find the best fit from that menu of things; smoking cessation, exercise on prescription, weight management and falls prevention. And so with the right amount of guidance and some incentives we have actually commissioned a range of schemes across the different PBC groups.' (PBC lead, site 8)

Despite these initiatives, practice-based commissioners were often considered tangential to the commissioning process, unaware of the WCC competencies, demands on PCTs including the Quality, Innovation, Productivity and Prevention (QIPP) initiative which required the NHS to make £20 billion of savings by 2015.

> 'There aren't clear commissioning principles embedded into the practice-based commissioning process, although there are in the PCT process. So that's the problem.' (PBC lead, site 5)

And, from another site:

> 'I have to say at the moment that recognition of the world class commissioning competence framework among practice-based commissioners is pretty low. I mean I'm sure they, I think they probably now know what we're talking about. Part of me thinks why on earth would we inflict the extraordinary degree of process that surrounds WCC on consortia?' (DPH, site 7)

PCT interviewees considered it important that practice-based commissioners developed skills in commissioning on a larger scale and in more complex areas. They also needed to develop strong business cases in the context of wider strategic priorities and a broader health agenda including commissioning through wider partnerships:

> 'And for me it's always been an issue with practice-based commissioning.... I went through five years of specialist training to come out as a commissioner about the needs of the population. Overnight we expected these people, whose whole training, whose whole raison d'être for getting out of bed in the morning is about the individual, and very few of them have got a mindset beyond that. So I think it's really, really difficult.' (DPH, site 2 in Marks et al., 2011c: 17)

This was reflected in a view that general practice had a limited appreciation of a health and wellbeing agenda:

> 'There's a barrier which is around a lack of understanding about what the wellbeing agenda is about.... there's still quite a large element of general practice that views public health and wellbeing in very traditional terms as being about the kind of old-fashioned health promotion and public health campaigns with posters on the walls and adverts telling people to do this and not do that and handing out leaflets at general practices and in pharmacies. And while that undoubtedly has a role it's really only a very, it's only a part, and you could say a small part of the way that we would want to go about health improvement in the city. So there is a barrier about their lack of a real understanding about the way that we want to address a health improvement agenda.' (DPH, site 7)

While it was argued that PBC needed to be involved in designing and contributing to health needs assessments, in general, their involvement in a wider health and wellbeing agenda was not well developed, with interests mainly focused on managing demand for acute care and reconfiguring pathways of care.

> 'Well theoretically you would say that they were heavily involved. In reality, I would say it's fairly minimal. I would say that most family doctor practices see health and wellbeing as a public health issue that's beyond their scope, and unless they're funded to get involved with it like providing screening for cardiovascular risk or providing long-term condition management for diabetes then I think most of them would see it as outside of their particular role.' (NED [non-executive director], site 7)

These problems were partly attributed to the nature of PBC. Many interviewees saw it as confused, a 'policy puzzle': governance tensions over the separation of commissioner and provider responsibilities were inherent to PBC (although some interviewees were confident that governance structures provided effective firewalls between the two roles). Complicated arrangements had been put in place in some areas to address this problem, such as setting up separate provider companies.

> 'There's a fundamental problem with practice-based commissioning in that you've got the seller if you like advising the buyer what to buy. Well, what would you advise them to buy?' (NED, site 7)

These conflicts were difficult to address, with GPs described as seeing their role mainly as providers.

> 'There's a whole lot of ... potential conflicts of interest really, and that's been one of the most extraordinary things to see, because people have had to excuse themselves from decisions because they're actually bidding for services as well. So it's a real sort of tangle of conflicts, I think.' (DPH, site 6)

Lessons from the research for public health in local government

Since April 2013, local authorities have taken on new public health responsibilities to be reflected not just through the deployment of a public health budget (transferred from the NHS and ring-fenced until 2016) but across the range of local authority services. The expectation is that local authorities will exert greater influence over the social determinants of health (or at least those amenable to local action); will be better able to address inequities in health, for which the Marmot Review (2010) provided a framework; and will promote better integration of health and social care through HWBs. For instance, examples of proposals for practical evidence-based interventions that local government could implement to address the social determinants of health and reduce health inequalities (British Academy, 2014) included the living wage, improving life chances in early childhood through integrated education centres, speed limits in residential areas, tackling health-related worklessness, participatory budgeting and building age-friendly communities. The aspiration expressed in WCC for PCTs to become 'community leaders' certainly seems unrealistic when compared with the already established leadership role of local government and their democratic mandate. Local authorities can build on their knowledge of local communities and community networks to reshape services and align initiatives across a wide range of commissioning strategies. The risk of identifying health and wellbeing with health care and with lifestyle interventions is less likely under the new arrangements and the sources of wellbeing can be influenced through local authorities' 'place-shaping' role. However, in the same way that, in the study, the financial crisis threatened preventive services in PCTs, so current reductions in local government funding are likely to lead to a focus on non-negotiable statutory requirements in local authorities and on the health and social care agenda. Just as many PCTs in the study identified commissioning for health and wellbeing with the sum total of their current activity, so local authorities may identify public health with the sum total of local authority activities. For different reasons, neither of these options is likely to promote investment in proactive identification of those at risk of premature mortality. While in the previous arrangements there were some opportunities for shifting NHS budgets and pathways of care towards prevention, given the potential return on investment for the NHS, CCGs are not currently charged with commissioning public health services and therefore may not prioritise them as part of the NHS budget.

—

There is scope in the new commissioning arrangements to further develop a participatory, community-based approach and increase the role of JSNAs in promoting transparency in decision making and priority setting. Perhaps the most significant aspect of the relocation of JSNAs to local authority HWBs is this increased scrutiny and transparency. The Local Government Association (Harding et al., 2011: 8) summed up the new context and the increased prominence of the JSNA:

> This backdrop will challenge most JSNAs to respond to the needs of changing audiences, greater political prominence and an environment of increased scrutiny, transparency and accountability. For example, commentators may look to JSNAs to provide a clearer rationale for hierarchy of need across the system, so driving strategic prioritisation and 'big picture' investment or disinvestment decisions.

CCGs have a duty to engage with the JSNA which should inform their commissioning decisions (as well as those of NHS England, responsible for commissioning local primary care services and for primary care contracts). As part of the public health responsibilities of local government, DsPH are to give support and advice to CCGs including for the development and implementation of the JSNA, which is likely to involve targeted activities to reduce health inequalities (a statutory requirement for CCGs). While local authorities can ask CCGs to account for commissioning priorities which do not reflect the JSNA, there are no sanctions in place. It remains to be seen how far CCGs will engage with the JSNA in practice and respond to its priorities − or whether the less engaged approach identified in the study will predominate.

Previous collaboration across PCTs and local authorities and successful joint DPH appointments are likely to influence progress in the new arrangements. While the JSNA has been strengthened, there are many other influences on commissioning and on priority setting, further discussed in Chapter Six.

Public health commissioning is taking place at a time when commissioning practice in local government is also changing, from a concern with procurement and performance management to a focus on place-based commissioning and on demonstrating value for money in achieving improved outcomes. This involves redesigning services and working with communities and agencies across the local area (Local Government Association, 2012). Commissioning mechanisms for improving outcomes might include 'pooling budgets, market management, partnership building, enhancing choice, harnessing voluntary and community resources and capacity, influencing partner spend and users decisions and behaviours' (Local Government Association, 2012: 3) – and mechanisms are not limited to the procurement of services. This demonstrates a broader approach to commissioning across a whole system than that typically reflected in NHS commissioning, which, despite the WCC initiative, often focused in practice on commissioning services and managing contracts in the acute sector.

The coalition government produced a set of three outcomes frameworks (for public health, the NHS and adult social care [Department of Health, 2012a, 2012b, 2012c]) which allow for authorities to benchmark their performance, set priorities and assess progress. In the case of the NHS, the outcomes framework also acts as an accountability mechanism with NHS England.

From a health and wellbeing perspective, a key question is the extent to which health and wellbeing is reflected in commissioning and priority setting across local authority directorates and CCGs. In addressing these issues, developing commissioning competencies, working through commissioning cycles, and understanding implications of the different approaches to health and wellbeing demonstrated in the study remain relevant.

Conclusions

While the importance of effective commissioning has been heightened due to unprecedented requirements for NHS efficiency gains, shortcomings of NHS commissioning arrangements over the previous two decades have been widely acknowledged and were reflected in two reports of the Health Committee, the first carried out under the Labour government (House of Commons Health Committee, 2010) and the second under the coalition government (House of Commons Health Committee, 2011). Although both reports focused on health care commissioning rather than preventive services, the problems identified were of wider application. These included a lack of skills, data analysis and effective management on the part of commissioners, and systemic problems arising from a lack of leverage over providers and conflicting system incentives, where acute sector activity was incentivised. These findings were reflected in an evaluation of the reforms instigated by the Labour government which noted that 'the reforms do not appear to comprise a coherent and mutually supportive set of arrangements, and appear "unbalanced" in that the "centre of gravity" favours suppliers over commissioners' (Millar et al., 2012: 7). While commissioning had been strengthened, professionalised even, through the core skills reflected in the commissioning competencies, resources and data were inadequate, partnerships were poorly developed and historical ways of working predominated (McCafferty et al., 2012). Also, as demonstrated in the study, the WCC assessment process and the profusion of targets were perceived as burdensome and worked against local decision making.

However, in the wake of the unexpected abolition of PCTs, it has been argued (NHS Confederation Primary Care Trust Network, 2011) that the performance of PCTs as commissioning organisations has been judged prematurely and that their performance was effective in relation to what they had been asked to deliver. Health outcomes had improved (although the health inequalities gap had widened), waiting time targets had been met and there were improvements in financial management. It was also pointed out that power imbalances between commissioners and providers were common and not unique to the English context.

Whatever the commissioning arrangements in force, there are advantages in commissioning focused on outcomes, a continuous commissioning cycle and the development of commissioning competencies. Despite the organisational upheavals and the abolition of WCC, NHS England's commissioning strategy (NHS England, 2014), for example, bears some resemblance to the original WCC competencies. However, it is also important to learn from the experience of PCTs as commissioning organisations. For example, a study on the implementation of WCC by PCTs (McCafferty et al., 2012) noted the importance of aligning policies, incentives and partnerships across the commissioning system, providing adequate funding and commissioning support, and relationship building in a context of increased organisational fragmentation. Such factors will continue to influence the chances of success of CCGs as new, relatively inexperienced, commissioners and of local authorities in their new and expanded public health role.

Notes
[1] See: http://hrep.lshtm.ac.uk/.

[2] See examples at: www.hcna.bham.ac.uk.

CHAPTER FOUR

Levers for change (1): governance arrangements

National governments have at their disposal a wide range of methods for realising policy intentions and for monitoring performance. These include policy guidelines and regulatory frameworks; standards and targets; and arrangements for audit and scrutiny. While governance arrangements of this kind are integral for ensuring accountability, the form they take is influenced by the approach adopted by the government in power to regulation and performance management. This affects the balance across regulatory and voluntary approaches, the extent to which legislation (including public health-related legislation) is adopted as an instrument of governance and the emphasis on self-assessment as opposed to centralised monitoring of organisations. As part of this, the landscape of standards and targets is liable to change, with shifting balances across central control of measurable targets and local flexibility, differences in the emphasis accorded to outcomes as opposed to process measures and varying recognition of partnership success as opposed to the success of single organisations. The transition, in 2010, from a Labour to a coalition government saw the deliberate dismantling of a complex and far-reaching system of governance arrangements, including those related to the NHS and local government. This affected the system of targets, incentives, monitoring and audit arrangements across the commissioning spectrum, including services for health improvement. Performance management of public services through a large number of explicit performance targets, was a characteristic feature of the former Labour government, sometimes described as a regime of 'targets and terror' (Bevan and Hood, 2006), although there was also a range of initiatives designed to support organisations in meeting targets. At the time of the study, improving health and narrowing the health gap were policy priorities, associated with directing resources towards disadvantaged groups and areas and reflected in a range of targets and performance management arrangements. These included the national targets for reducing inequalities, departmental public service agreements (PSAs), objectives in *Tackling health inequalities: A programme for action* (Department of Health, 2003a), the world class commissioning (WCC) assurance framework (Department of Health,

2008a, 2009a), and the 'Vital Signs' of the Annual Operating Framework for the NHS (Department of Health, 2008c). Reducing inequalities was also a mandatory indicator for targets agreed by local partnerships.

This chapter explores the influence of governance arrangements on decision making related to addressing health inequalities and promoting health and wellbeing at the time of the study, with a particular emphasis on performance assessment measures and the extent to which they were aligned across different agencies. The chapter begins by outlining the context for these governance arrangements, before describing how they influenced decision making in practice. It also illustrates broader questions over the effectiveness of approaches to performance management and their relevance to public health commissioning following the Health and Social Care Act 2012.

Governance arrangements in context

While governance arrangements are intended to support decision making which reflects underlying principles, they may not be well aligned, they may be associated with incentives which conflict, or certain elements – such as financial targets – may dominate at the expense of core values. Their effectiveness in achieving the aims of government policy as well as their relevance for specific policy priorities, such as the prevention of ill health, remain important questions for policy makers.

While performance management arrangements comprise systems for measuring performance and are associated with penalties and rewards, questions over what constitutes appropriate indicators for performance, the hazards of poorly designed performance management systems and the impact on outcomes of specific arrangements, such as targets, have been the subject of extensive study (Smith, 1995). Research studies have investigated the extent to which a target culture encourages various 'gaming' strategies (Bevan and Hood, 2006) and whether effective anti-gaming strategies are in place to prevent them (Hood, 2006). A target culture has also been associated with a panoply of other potential problems such as 'tunnel vision'; 'hitting the target and missing the point'; lack of innovation; 'cream skimming'; 'short termism'; and neglect of the wider purpose and value of the organisation (Goddard et al., 2000). It is also recognised that explicit targets may be ill suited to complex and multifactorial problems such as tackling health inequalities or obesity, which need concerted action across agencies (Blackman et al., 2006; Butland et al., 2007). Moreover, as Wismar et al. (2008) argue, managers are more likely to concentrate their effort on areas over which they have greatest control. This works against a focus on 'wicked issues' such as inequalities, which can only be tackled through collaboration across sectors over the longer term. Conversely, however, it is argued that targets can serve a useful purpose, providing a measurable indicator of an organisation's performance and fostering service improvement. It is also argued that involving stakeholders in developing indicators can improve the effectiveness of performance management arrangements (Mannion and Davies, 2008). These themes were reflected in an extensive programme of research on managing public service performance, funded through the Economic and Social Research Council (2004–10).[1]

Governance arrangements also influence the nature of incentives (Davies et al., 2005), further discussed in Chapter Five. National and local financial (and other) incentives may be put in place in order to meet standards and targets, with payments made if certain targets are reached. Conversely, penalties may result from failures in performance. In addition to debates over the effectiveness of targets or over the optimum balance to be achieved across locally selected targets and national priorities, the study raised specific questions over the extent to which performance management regimes and targets succeeded in prioritising health and wellbeing in practice, or whether a hierarchy of targets prevailed.

As indicated in Chapter Two, organisations act within a framework for corporate governance which incorporates systems for audit, risk management and regulation. For primary care trusts (PCTs) at the time of the study, these systems reflected an increasing number of contractual arrangements as a result of market-related reforms, extensive monitoring through independent regulators, numerous targets and a duty of partnership working, also associated with centralised targets and assessment. New developments during the period of the study included the implementation of the annual comprehensive area assessment (CAA) in 2009, the Care Quality Commission (CQC), also in 2009, the WCC assurance framework in 2007, and a new performance framework (Vital Signs) in 2008, as part of the Annual Operating Framework for the NHS. The CAA was a coordinated performance framework for local authorities (working alone and in partnership), focused on outcomes and on citizen and community perspectives. 'Direction of travel' and local use of resources were assessed and scored. These changes were interrelated so that, for example, assessments from WCC informed Audit Commission assessments of local use of resources, and partnerships were assessed through WCC and the CAA.

Boards were accountable for the effective governance of their organisations, for formulating strategy and assuring that systems of control were in place. The complex governance landscape for NHS organisations at the time of the study was reflected in *The healthy NHS board: Principles for good governance* (NHS National Leadership Council, 2010) which aimed to describe 'enduring principles of high quality governance, which transcend immediate policy imperatives and the more pressing features of the current health care environment' (p. 6). It pointed out the importance of understanding the policy, economic and legislative context, and the complex accountability arrangements between central bodies, independent regulators and NHS boards. The organisational landscape, spanning public, private and voluntary organisations also needed to be understood.

As described in more detail in the following section, the health and wellbeing agenda was subject to a bewildering array of performance assessment measures at the time of the study, including cross-cutting PSA targets for government departments, shared priorities and local area agreements (LAAs), implemented across England from 2008. (Both LAAs and local strategic partnerships [LSPs] originated with the Neighbourhood Renewal Strategy.) The context was that of a national audit regime based on top-down performance measurement with strong managerial incentives, involving Strategic Health Authorities (SHAs) and regional government offices (both since abolished). The early period of the study saw major developments in regulatory arrangements and the end of the study saw their subsequent abolition, reflecting a dramatic change of emphasis in the management of public services.

Governance arrangements in commissioning organisations

The governance arrangements that obtained in PCTs at the time of the study are briefly outlined to provide a context for the views of commissioners presented in this chapter. Although the coalition government implemented major changes in commissioning organisations and in performance management arrangements, questions over the extent to which aspects of performance management regimes can act as barriers or enablers for the health and wellbeing agenda are of wider relevance. In the same way, views over incentives which flowed from these governance arrangements provide an insight into the impact of incentives on commissioning practice.

At the time of the study, PCT boards had collective responsibility for performance and were accountable to the Department of Health through SHAs; to Parliament through independent regulators (the

Healthcare Commission [replaced by the CQC in April 2009] and the Audit Commission); and to local populations through local authority overview and scrutiny committees (OSCs). Accountability for contributing to partnerships and shared targets was assessed at the time of the study through the annual CAA (carried out by the Audit Commission from 2009) as well as by SHAs through the WCC process and by regional government offices (GOs), through three-year LAAs. These were developed through LSPs as the delivery plan for the local authority Sustainable Community Strategy. The annual health check carried out by the former Healthcare Commission, and then through the CQC, was considered key to 'good governance' (Storey et al., 2008). However, as discussed in Chapter Three, the WCC assurance process also proved increasingly influential over the course of the study, with PCTs reshaping their organisational structures and governance arrangements to reflect their role as commissioning organisations. OSCs at the time of the study had little involvement in scrutinising progress on the health and wellbeing agenda but focused on health services and issues brought to councillors' attention by members of the public. There were few links across the various subgroups of scrutiny committees to reflect a cross-cutting health and wellbeing agenda and, in general, the scrutiny function appeared to play a minor role in governance arrangements of PCTs. The following section briefly describes the complex framework of standards, targets and regulation, with particular reference to their relevance to health and wellbeing.

Standards related to promoting health

Standards related to promoting health can be included as part of the following:

- national service frameworks (NSFs), which arose from the 1997 White Paper *The new NHS: Modern, dependable* (Secretary of State for Health, 1997);
- evidence-based guidelines produced by the National Institute for Health and Care Excellence (NICE) on specific topics;
- national topic-based strategies, such as the obesity strategy (Department of Health, 2008b, 2011e), tobacco strategy (Department of Health, 2011d) and alcohol strategy (Secretary of State for the Home Department, 2012);
- core standards (assessed annually at the time of the project through the annual health check and, since 2009, through the CQC for hospitals, care homes and care services).

NSFs (nine at the time of writing) were launched in 1998 and are intended to provide long-term strategies and clear quality requirements for improving care. They set national standards, identify key interventions and measurable goals, and provide a timeline for implementation. They are updated and reported on (although at variable intervals). Many of the NSFs include preventive components, for example, standards one and two of the NSF for coronary heart disease relate to reducing heart disease in the population and reducing smoking. Some monitoring of national strategies was carried out via the improvement reviews of the former Healthcare Commission, including tobacco control, diabetes and sexual health services (Healthcare Commission, 2007a, 2007b, 2007c). However, NSF recommendations and milestones for prevention were not routinely performance managed or prioritised by commissioners in the study: neither were NSFs systematically reflected through the performance management system. Moreover, there has often been a time lag between identifying public health problems and developing national strategy. It has been pointed out, for example, that the national strategy for obesity did not appear until 2008, while the target for reducing obesity, set in 1992, was dropped in 1997 and did not reappear in PSAs until 2004 (Healthcare Commission and Audit Commission, 2008). Recent topic-based strategies, such as for tobacco control (Department of Health, 2011d) include 'national ambitions' for specific reductions in smoking rates but these are not tied into a performance management framework.

The Centre for Public Health Excellence at NICE develops public health intervention guidance and broader public health programme guidance (with 52 topics included at the time of writing). Developed in the context of a broad conceptual framework for public health (Kelly et al., 2009), NICE provides guidance for evidence-based interventions and implementation strategies of local partnerships. NICE guidance has also been provided for local government and, in particular, for those involved in health and wellbeing boards (HWBs). Seventeen briefings have been prepared to date (including tobacco, workplace health, physical activity, health inequalities and population health, alcohol, behaviour change and return on investment) with others in development. Each briefing includes costs and savings, examples of action plans and support tools.[2] NICE has also developed 'quality standards' across health, public health and social care, based on the latest evidence and best practice with the first public health quality standards, based on NICE public health guidance, developed from May 2013. Initial quality standards are focused on reducing tobacco use in the community, preventing harmful alcohol use, and strategies to prevent obesity in adults and children.

The NHS has a legal obligation to meet NICE guidelines. However, public health guidance often lacks the specificity of clinical guidelines and there is no legal obligation for local authorities to implement it, despite evidence of cost-effectiveness.

At the time of the study, annual health checks were carried out by the Healthcare Commission (from 2006) and, from 2009, by the CQC. Healthcare Commission checks were based on 'core' and 'developmental' standards across seven domains, including safety, clinical- and cost-effectiveness and patient focus (Department of Health, 2004). Providing a common set of requirements, as well as a way of measuring performance, they constituted a key assurance process for PCTs at the time of the study: PCTs were required to demonstrate compliance with core standards and respond to any shortcomings. There was also an assessment of the extent to which PCTs had achieved their targets.

Good governance in PCTs was sometimes equated with meeting these standards. The annual health check included core standards for public health, which occupied a separate (seventh) domain. It has been pointed out (Healthcare Commission and Audit Commission, 2008: 41) that, internationally, the Healthcare Commission was the only regulator with statutory responsibilities to assess health care organisations in relation to public health delivery – a feature, it is argued, that proved beneficial for local health improvement. The aim of the public health domain was that 'programmes and services are designed and delivered in collaboration with all the relevant organisations and communities to promote, protect and improve the health of the population served and reduce health inequalities between different population groups and areas' (Department of Health, 2004: 34). One of the core standards (C23) was that

> health care organisations have systematic and managed disease prevention and health promotion programmes which meet the requirements of the NSFs and national plans with particular regard to reducing obesity through action on nutrition and exercise, smoking, substance misuse and sexually transmitted infections. (Department of Health, 2004: 34)

There were also a number of developmental standards which implied anticipatory governance, taking into account 'emerging policies and knowledge on public health issues'.

This emphasis on assessment of public health standards was short lived, however. As part of the changes that have taken place since the replacement of the Healthcare Commission by the CQC, public health has receded from view in the assessment process. The focus is on the quality and safety of care offered by providers (Care Quality Commission, 2013) rather than on including standards expected from commissioners of care, and there are no equivalent public health standards included as part of formal NHS assessment procedures.

Targets and performance management regimes

The system of targets put in place through the Labour government was highly complex (see Box 4.1) and was intended as part of a framework of reforms 'with the right incentives, levers and enablers' (HM Treasury, 2007a: 3). There were national and local targets; some were negotiable and others non-negotiable; they emanated from different sources (which were not always aligned); they sometimes overlapped; and were subject to different inspection regimes. They were also associated with different rewards and penalties.

Box 4.1: Targets for health and wellbeing

Public service agreements (1998–2010)

PSAs (with 600 targets) were established following the 1998 comprehensive spending review (CSR) which set three-year budgets for government ministries; targets were reduced in subsequent CSRs. A reduced number of 30 PSAs emerged from the Treasury's 2007 CSR (HM Treasury, 2007b). PSAs 12, 18 and 19 were of particular relevance to health and wellbeing and PSA18 included increased life expectancy; reducing premature mortality between the Spearhead groups (the most disadvantaged fifth of local authorities) and the national average; reducing smoking prevalence; increasing independence; and offering psychological therapies. The national inequalities target had formed part of the PSAs for 2002, 2004 and 2007 and was reaffirmed as part of PSA18 where all-age all-cause mortality [AAACM] was used as a proxy measure for the life expectancy element of the target, although the 2010 national inequalities target, with its emphasis on narrowing the gap, also remained in force. AAACM was also reflected in the NHS Operating Framework (Department of Health, 2009c) (see Vital Signs) and as part of the NIS, as indicator N120 in the category 'Adult Health and Well Being'. Encouraging partnerships was built into the structure of LAAs and PSAs

---

and reflected in assessment procedures. There was a combination of negotiable and non-negotiable targets and 'floor targets' agreed for disadvantaged areas or groups where there was weak delivery.

The National Indicator Set (2007–10) and local area agreements (2004–10)
The 2007 CSR also announced a new NIS for monitoring the performance of local authorities and local authority partnerships in relation to the priorities of the CSR and, from 2009, the NIS was used to monitor the performance of local authorities and partnerships through the annual CAA. LSPs could choose a maximum of 35 local improvement targets from the NIS (and could also choose additional local targets, in line with the findings of local JSNAs, which were then negotiated with GOs). Developed through LSPs, LAAs were the vehicle for delivering these targets. They were made a statutory obligation in 2008 and rolled out across England. Achievements were rewarded through an area-based grant thus giving local councils more control over how to distribute funding. The focus on LAAs underlined the importance attached to the joint setting and delivery of targets and of partnership working to deliver better outcomes in both health and social care. Performance was monitored by the former GOs in the regions.

National inequalities targets (2002–10)
The NHS Plan (Secretary of State for Health, 2000) introduced the first ever health inequalities targets for England. The national inequalities target was, by 2010, to reduce inequalities in health outcomes by 10% as measured by life expectancy at birth and infant mortality. This target was underpinned by two more detailed objectives:

*   starting with local authorities, by 2010 to reduce by at least 10% the gap in life expectancy at birth between the fifth of areas with the worst health and deprivation indicators and the population as a whole;
*   starting with children under one year, by 2010 to reduce by at least 10% the gap in mortality between the routine and manual group and the population as a whole.

Reducing health inequalities and increasing life expectancy were mandatory health outcomes for all PCTs, as part of WCC.

Vital Signs
The 2010/11 Annual Operating Framework for the NHS in England continued to adopt Vital Signs, first introduced in the 2008/9 operating framework, as the basis for assessing health outcomes and health care (Department of Health, 2009c). PCTs reflected these priorities in their local plans (Annual Operating Plans). The 2008/9 framework encouraged PCTs to deliver jointly agreed outcomes through LAAs and their own operational plans. Vital Signs had a three-tier approach:

national headline priorities; national priorities for local delivery (associated with 17 indicators) where there was some flexibility about local targets; and local priorities associated with 33 indicators, although PCTs were not limited to these. There were five headline national priorities: improving cleanliness and reducing health care associated infections; improving access through the 18-week referral to treatment pledge and improving access to GP surgeries; keeping adults and children well, improving their health and reducing health inequalities; improving patient experience, staff satisfaction and engagement; and preparing to respond in a state of emergency. These were associated with 13 indicators.

Where there was overlap with indicators in the NIS, these could also be pursued through an LAA and there were 31 indicators in Vital Signs which formed part of the NIS. While local priorities were to be determined and set locally in consultation with patients, public, staff, and in accordance with the findings of JSNAs and agreed with partners, there was no performance management role through the Department of Health.

Key agreements and targets included three-year PSAs, focused on outcomes. These originated in the 1998 comprehensive spending review (CSR), and set out key cross-departmental priorities for public spending in order to hold public services to account, underpinned by a delivery agreement. LAAs were the delivery mechanism for 35 locally selected joint targets agreed across a local authority area and approved by GOs. There were two national health inequalities targets, agreed in 2002; the National Indicator Set (NIS) (198 indicators) for local authorities, dating from 2007 (Department for Communities and Local Government, 2007); and the Annual Operating Framework for PCTs, which included Vital Signs (from 2008). Following the 2007 CSR, a more streamlined approach was adopted – PSAs were reduced from 145 to 30, for example, along with attempts to better align performance regimes.

It is important to emphasise that health and wellbeing and health inequalities were included throughout this complex monitoring process, forming part of three PSAs (12, 18 and 19), Vital Signs and the NIS. As mentioned in Chapter Three, reducing health inequalities and increasing life expectancy were mandatory outcomes for all PCTs as part of WCC, and LAAs reflected the importance attached to joint working across local authorities and PCTs for better outcomes for both health and social care.

Annual reports from the Healthcare Commission summarised progress against targets including health inequalities, and against planned performance, as included in PCT local plans. The Audit

Commission audited local councils through the CAA, working with other inspectorates. Through local auditors, it also audited PCTs in relation to key risks and their effectiveness and efficiency in using public funds, producing an annual Auditors' Local Evaluation (ALE letter). Auditors considered how well organisations were managing and using their resources to deliver value for money and better and sustainable outcomes through a 'use of resources framework' (introduced in May 2008). The framework was structured into three themes: sound and strategic financial management; strategic commissioning and good governance; and the effective management of natural resources, assets and people. From 2009, the use of resources framework formed part of the short-lived CAA and other performance management frameworks. Crucially, partners would be held collectively to account for their performance and the extent to which they achieved aims for the local area by main public sector inspectorates working more closely together, as opposed to the previous system of the Audit Commission performance managing councils through the Comprehensive Performance Assessment process. This would help assess whether investment as a whole was aligned with the needs of the community. Local scrutiny was provided through local authority OSCs.

Despite attempts at streamlining, a large number of indicators remained (although only a minority were associated with targets/ minimum standards), often in the form of 'legacy indicators', sub-indicators or performance objectives under headline targets. There were 157 indicators for the 30 PSAs, for example, plus legacy indicators and each organisation had targets of its own. Local authorities were also monitored on all 198 indicators of the NIS (Department for Communities and Local Government, 2007). It was argued that while the NIS was introduced with the intention of streamlining local performance management, new indicators were simply added to existing measures (Gash et al., 2008). Despite similar attempts to streamline targets in NHS Vital Signs, the reduced numbers did not represent the whole picture given a range of pre-existing commitments and priorities.

While targets did interrelate (with the same targets appearing in different frameworks where actions required cooperation across both the NHS and local authorities, for example), the existence of separate streams of indicators performance managed through local government and the NHS and the sheer number of targets involved, created a risk that overarching cross-cutting targets would become displaced by a focus on detailed organisation-specific targets, where there was greater control by the organisations concerned.

There was widespread criticism of the target regime as a whole as too complicated, not well enough aligned across the various monitoring agencies and time consuming. Research carried out by the Institute for Government (Gash et al., 2008) showed that some targets were widely considered unachievable within a three-year time frame (such as reductions in all-age all-cause mortality [AAACM] rates); others were difficult for some areas to achieve (such as the teenage pregnancy target); baseline data were often lacking; and some indicators were unclear or poorly designed. It was also difficult to prioritise across different targets. The relationships between PSAs, the NIS, Departmental Strategic Objectives and Vital Signs were so complex that various mapping exercises were carried out to try to clarify the arrangements. Despite high hopes for the LAA, it was noted by the then chair of the Local Government Association that 'what was conceived as a framework for joint working, energising innovative working between partners and reinvigorated governance has become bogged down in bureaucratic process and multiple targets' (Improvement and Development Agency, 2007: 2). Splits were described between strategic priority setting through local authority Sustainable Community Strategies on the one hand and the process for deciding LAAs on the other. Moreover, despite being intended as a route for local autonomy and devolved control, some saw statutory LAAs as further examples of top-down control, with less room for manoeuvre than anticipated. It was argued that a 'delivery chain' model designed to improve performance had taken over 'local place shaping' (Improvement and Development Agency, 2007). There was also a lack of alignment across LAAs and WCC outcomes, so that, for example, a reduction in AAACM was mandatory for PCTs but adopted by only 88 LSPs (Audit Commission, 2010).

Overlapping layers of standards and targets in health improvement, combined with inconsistent approaches to priority setting led to confusion. For example, fuel poverty was a priority in *Tackling health inequalities: A programme for action* (Department of Health, 2003a) but not included in the public health White Paper, *Choosing health* (Secretary of State for Health, 2004). There was also some confusion about the status of health improvement issues not included as PSAs. In any event, policy priorities were not always reflected in local implementation strategies.

The coalition government set about dismantling the array of targets and other centralised performance management arrangements. It abandoned the PSAs, the LAAs and the CAA. It replaced the NIS for local authorities with an agreed single list of Whitehall data requirements for local government. GOs were closed. Finally, the performance assessment system reflected in the WCC initiative was discontinued.

While the complexity and overlapping nature of the targets is evident, the consistency of concern to address inequalities through the range of policies, monitoring and performance management procedures over a 13-year period was also lost. This had given rise to England's reputation as having the most systematic approach to addressing inequalities 'with a target which is arguably the toughest anywhere in the world, and which has received international plaudits' (House of Commons Health Committee, 2009: 6). However, it is also the case that while life expectancy improved over the period, the health gap did not, reflecting the scale of interventions required, the cumulative nature of health inequalities and their links with wider socioeconomic inequalities (Mackenbach, 2010).

Views from the study

The study assessed views of how the system of performance management related to health and wellbeing through three routes: a national survey, national and regional focus groups and local interviewee accounts. Knowledge of performance management was mainly limited to PCTs (with the exception of local involvement networks [LINks], which had responsibility for reviewing the annual health check) and few practice-based commissioners were aware of the detail of performance management systems.

While interviewees approved, in principle, of performance management for health and wellbeing, as it was a route for monitoring progress, they pointed out numerous inadequacies in the system. The national survey located views of performance management arrangements in context through asking respondents to rate how supportive each of a range of factors was for health and wellbeing (Table 4.1). This demonstrates the relatively minor role played by various performance management regimes in encouraging an emphasis on health and wellbeing, as compared, for example, with board values. Only 14.9% of respondents strongly supported the role of current performance management systems in this respect, compared with 63.2% who supported board values. It also showed the relatively greater role accorded to the LAA and the CAA, compared with the annual health check. This underlines the importance accorded to local partnerships for furthering a public health agenda.

Given the ubiquity and complexity of targets, it is not surprising that strong views were expressed both in focus groups and interviewee accounts. Interviewees reflected a range of views on targets, their benefits and limitations. Most commissioners considered performance

Table 4.1: Factors influencing support for health and wellbeing

	Strongly support	Quite strongly support	Medium support	Weak support	Very weak support	N/A	Total no. responses
Board values	63.2% (55)	25.3% (22)	11.5% (10)	0	0	0	87
Current performance management systems	14.9% (13)	32.2% (28)	34.5% (30)	12.6% (11)	4.6% (4)	1.1% (1)	87
Financial allocations	23.9% (21)	17.0% (15)	12.5% (11)	18.2% (16)	26.1% (23)	2.3% (2)	88
Annual health check	16.1% (14)	34.5% (30)	26.4% (23)	17.2% (15)	5.7% (5)	0	87
Comprehensive area assessment	18.4% (16)	47.1% (41)	20.7% (18)	9.2% (8)	3.4% (3)	1.1% (1)	87
PBC priorities	8.2% (7)	24.7% (21)	22.4% (19)	35.3% (30)	9.4% (8)	0	85
PCT prioritisation methods	27.6% (24)	37.9% (33)	19.5% (17)	11.5% (10)	2.3% (2)	1.1% (1)	87
LAAs	20.9% (18)	57.0% (49)	19.8% (17)	1.2% (1)	1.2% (1)	0	86
Public involvement strategies	9.2% (8)	36.8% (32)	34.5% (30)	14.9% (13)	3.4% (3)	1.1% (1)	87

Source: Marks et al. (2011a: 56)

management regimes as a driver for improvement for PCTs. However, these systems did not apply to GPs, as the GP contract was mainly monitored through the Quality and Outcomes Framework (QOF), the pay-for-performance element of the general medical services (GMS) contract (see Chapter Five).

There was general agreement, expressed in the majority of sites, that the system was overloaded with targets and that new targets were just added on to existing ones. One interviewee noted:

> 'I think the problem is there's just so many of the blooming things. You know, there's so many Vital Signs, and no matter how many new initiatives we get, they add to the existing list of targets that we have, rather than actually reduce them.' (DPH, site 6)

Questions were raised over the extent to which indicators supported longer-term outcomes, whether health and wellbeing indicators were prioritised and over inadequate alignment across performance management systems. A key issue was that a short-term target culture could work against a stewardship role and the assessment of longer-term risks to public health and gaps in service provision:

> 'But the bit that's missing is the kind of due diligence, the bit that in twenty years' time ... they'd say why on earth didn't you notice that and do something about it? And the answer of course is it wasn't a target. Or it wasn't required of us.' (National focus group)

The annual financial planning round discouraged a focus on improving health over the longer term in favour of investments where payback was more immediate:

> 'The problem we have at the moment in having to do the yearly cycle means that some of the things, if they're not going to payback within year two, then you very quickly lose interest in investing in them because something that's going to payback this year is actually going to be far more of a draw to the finance team.' (PEC chair, site 10)

As demonstrated in previous studies (Hunter and Marks, 2005; Blackman et al., 2006), not all targets were subject to the same level of scrutiny. Despite national targets for narrowing the health gap, and an emphasis on reducing health inequalities in national guidance and through performance management frameworks, this proved no guarantee for their being prioritised in practice. Over 80% of PCT interviewees considered that their focus remained on central priorities, the 'must be dones', which reflected government priorities: the control of health care acquired infections; an 18-week limit on referral to treatment time; Accident and Emergency waits under four hours; and the duty to remain in financial balance.

> 'The reality is that public health has been squeezed because all of the targets and all of the performance measures have been about delivering health care against a massive deficit in the budget.' (NED [non-executive director], site 7)

These targets were reflected in performance management arrangements with the SHA as well as with external regulatory bodies and were non-negotiable. They also influenced spending priorities. SHAs were described as being largely focused on central priorities, which did not always align with local priorities and targets, LAAs or with the public health agenda. This was the case, despite inclusion of health improvement targets in performance management systems:

> 'I think it's very frustrating that some of the high level targets around all-age all-cause mortality, IMD [Index of Multiple Deprivation], life expectancy are all supposed to be very, very important but actually when the strategic health authority comes to visit they're mostly interested in 18-week waits.... I'm glad that we do have priorities for performance management, and I'm a real strong advocate for if they're the right targets then if we deliver on it we'll have the impact that we desire. But it does sometimes feel, as I said, like we've got them but actually people aren't particularly interested in them.' (DPH, site 8)

Moreover, electoral cycles predisposed to short-term targets, and only some targets were considered 'career limiting'.

> 'I just think the realpolitik is what am I going to get sacked over, failure to deliver smoking cessation or failure to deliver the 18-week target? When smoking cessation has the same value and priority as the other 152 targets then it'll get the same emphasis. Have you heard of a chief executive in the NHS being sacked for failing to deliver smoking cessation? Have you heard of them being sacked for failing to deliver 18 weeks?' (Director of strategy, site 2)

Trajectories agreed with the SHA could prove unrealistic in practice. Two PCTs gave examples of challenging smoking cessation targets which had been met, but the same target had been maintained, even though this would now be more difficult to achieve. Performance management regimes were also criticised by commissioners for encouraging issues to be considered in isolation and, in particular, for focusing on process measures and activity rather than on outcomes. Measurement of processes was often appropriate for secondary care activity but much less so for health and wellbeing. Links between processes and outcomes were not always clear: as one example, measuring progress towards meeting the target for four-week quitters or 13-week quitters for smoking cessation was not a valid indicator of improved outcomes. Neither were the processes for achieving the targets under commissioner control: one interviewee described this in terms of the AAACM target:

> 'Now, if you look at targets, for example, for all-age all-cause mortality, it's very different because ... you can't manage the process of reducing all-age all-cause mortality in anything like the same way that you can manage the process of waiting times for surgery. You know, you just can't say right well if we invest a million pounds in this it will bring it down by this much or if we invest a million pounds there it will bring it down by that much and therefore that's what we'll do.' (DPH, site 7)

It was argued that targets should be outcome-based rather than focused on processes, and that indicators should be developed in conjunction with frontline staff and users.

In five case study sites (including the two highest performing sites), targets were viewed in a different light. It was argued that, for high-performing organisations, targets should be a by-product of culture, systems and processes, rather than the sole focus of endeavour. What lay behind the target needed to be understood in order to avoid 'hitting the target but missing the point'. Only by performing well against targets in general should organisations be given the freedom to innovate. Some interviewees emphasised that the health and wellbeing agenda was an 'earned agenda', dependent on the achievement of financial balance and delivering key targets. This was reflected across both practice-based commissioning (PBC) and PCT interviewees:

> 'Where you have a culture in performance, you keep financial balance, you deliver the targets and that's what gives you the platform from which to practice the public health agenda ... [it] gives you the licence to do the rest.' (PCT chief executive, site 3)

This could also mean that prioritisation of public health investment was always liable to deferral in the face of other priorities.

Views over the alignment of performance management regimes

PCTs typically tried to achieve alignment across the range of targets, including WCC health outcomes, LAAs and Vital Signs but this was not always considered possible as NHS targets were not the same as

LAAs. QOF targets also differed from PCT targets. There were also challenges in achieving alignment across LAAs where PCTs spanned a number of local authorities. While there had been some improvements in alignment across the regulators, it was argued that alignment was more evident at a strategic level than at the 'sharp end' of assessment. Concern over a lack of alignment between SHAs and GOs was of concern to commissioners in all case study sites. One interviewee commented:

> 'So Monitor, the Care Quality Commission, the strategic health authority and the Audit Commission, and they all have very, very different agendas, all of which impact on different bits of the health care and indeed social care system, and indeed more broadly into the sort of partnership agenda with comprehensive area assessment, and they are aligned in the very broadest most strategic sense, but when it comes to checking things at the sharp end, of course they don't join up.' (Director of strategy, site 7)

The existence of an intermediate layer of performance management, in the form of the SHA, was a major difference between the NHS and local government, and this was reflected in difficulties over negotiating local targets. Lack of alignment between PCT and SHA priorities was seen as a barrier in half the sites. Failure to integrate performance management regimes was commonly cited as a governance issue and reflected in difficulties in monitoring LAAs. One interviewee commented:

> 'I think the SHA struggled to understand the local area agreement, have failed to actually integrate its performance management into their performance management systems and haven't even managed to turn on the government office computer that we can monitor our own LAA through.... So it is not joined up, the LAA are monitored down the one side, and in fact we were filling [in] CAA monitoring and LAA monitoring stuff recently, at the same time as filling in exactly the same forms, with slightly different data for world class commissioning outcomes – I mean what a nonsense, no integration across. No integration across government office and SHA.' (PCT chief executive, site 2)

Interviewees also commented on the lack of alignment between ambitious SHA indicators and targets and those negotiated with GOs and reflected in the LAA. As a result, PCTs often ended up attempting to renegotiate one common target where councils were unwilling to sign up to 'undeliverable targets' or working towards two different targets with dual reporting. It was pointed out, for example, that Vital Signs trajectories were 'refreshed' at a different time from the LAA indicators, which could create problems: one interviewee described how a range of targets could be related to one indicator, depending on whether it formed part of the LAA or of Vital Signs. It was argued that where Vital Signs did not overlap with the WCC strategic priorities that there was less focus on them, simply because penalties were less severe.

At a local level, however, there were examples of joint approaches to performance management across PCTs and local authorities. In one site, some performance management staff were paid by the PCT but managed by the council. Some PCTs had developed web-based systems for monitoring strategic objectives, including partnership objectives, which were shared with the local authority and which, it was argued, helped to keep a focus on the health and wellbeing agenda.

Views of regulation and monitoring of partnerships

PCT commissioners from all sites commented on the CAA, which was viewed as potentially encouraging a focus on health and wellbeing for non-NHS organisations, increasing the emphasis on health and wellbeing within partnerships and reducing the tendency for health to be perceived solely as PCT business. The consensus was that it would have a positive impact on encouraging joined-up assessment of partnerships. Interviewees in three sites considered that the assessment process would encourage partner agencies to work together for common outcomes. All partners across a local area would need to consider how their services could improve the health and wellbeing of their local population:

> 'I hope it will have the effect of making the local authority more aware of its health and wellbeing responsibilities and more willing to cooperate with the PCT in delivering those responsibilities. Clearly there's a very explicit focus in the comprehensive area assessment on the way in which local organisations work together, so I guess it will make us consider that in more specific detail.' (DPH, site 7)

Some focus group participants considered that a new kind of accountability was emerging through the CAA which would assess whether investment was aligned with the needs of the community. It was also argued by local interviewees that the CAA would focus on the overall impact of partnerships on the local population rather than on the performance of individual organisations. This would encourage a shift to partnership working:

> 'Everyone will realise that they're dependent on each other in a way that they haven't been before in terms of partnership working, in order to attain their rating [so] that it will actually make people work together for the better.... It will make partnership very much more real.' (OSC chair, site 10)

There were some less positive views: a few interviewees were concerned that the CAA could become an additional and separate burden and that it would prove difficult to meet the assessment criteria. Others argued that the CAA was perceived as council led:

> 'Everybody at the PCT today will tell you in an instant what world class commissioning is, what their part to play is in it. Half of them wouldn't know what CAA stood for to be honest because it's not seen as relevant.' (Director of strategy, site 3)

Interviewees from the OSC and the voluntary and community sector (VCS) also questioned the extent to which the public or scrutiny committees would be involved, whether public views would be incorporated in the assessments and if the CAA would assess how well public agencies engaged with the voluntary sector. However, the fact that the results of the assessment were publicly available was considered an important public resource, providing comparative information about services and about performance. It would also be used as part of WCC assessments, described as 'one of our key measures of development and improvement'.

Interviewees and focus groups expressed optimism over the potential role of LAAs to make public health a shared priority for wider partnerships and to shift the focus away from the current emphasis on organisational governance towards partnership governance focused on a local area, or the 'governance of place', a topic which was reflected through the 'Total Place' initiative until 2010 (HM Treasury and

Department for Communities and Local Government, 2010) and subsequently through community-based budgets, introduced by the coalition government.

LAAs could make public health a shared priority for the wider partnership and therefore encourage improvement through partnership working. Negotiations over LAAs also involved debates over governance and accountability for achieving health outcomes. However, concerns were also expressed that LAAs could become reduced to debates about indicators and the process of measurement and were not locally owned:

> 'I think there's been so much top-down effort put into them, that they're almost guaranteed to be delivered by the time that they're actually put in place, and therefore it just feels like a grant condition, rather than actually something which is genuinely owned.' (National focus group)

Despite policy intentions to reduce the number of national targets, and focus on targets which were more locally relevant, there was pressure to include specific targets and measures in LAAs, some of which were considered unachievable. Tensions remained between national targets and local priorities and the inability to target investment to address local problems. A focus group participant noted that, 'what we were doing was in line with the national targets, but it wasn't in line with the scale of the problem on our patch at all'.

As already mentioned, governance of partnerships was undermined by constant reorganisations as each shift in structure meant that governance structures had to be reorganised. A lack of coterminosity across PCTs and local authorities in some areas meant limited PCT capacity to support partnerships, align priorities or support different LAAs within each of a number of boroughs. Large geographical areas also made it difficult for the VCS to coordinate their response and they lacked the resources to cover the costs of VCS involvement. The lack of an umbrella VCS body could make it difficult to coordinate views.

This analysis reveals conflicting views about targets. Clearly, interviewees felt that there were far too many targets, they were not well aligned and that the business of monitoring targets was becoming an end in itself. In relation to health promotion, a profusion of targets did not mean that they were prioritised in practice and, moreover, health promotion did not lend itself to target setting in the same way as process indicators, such as four-hour waits in Accident and Emergency. Outcomes were difficult to measure and were not under the control of a single organisation. However, the importance of partnerships for the health and wellbeing agenda was reflected in support for jointly agreed LAAs and the former CAA. It was also the case that targets, if enforced, were considered to drive improvement. Addressing health inequalities and improving health were proving difficult to prioritise, however, even with targets in place. The question, therefore, remains whether they will slip further down the priority scale without incentives in the form of performance management.

However, there was an important exception to the rather mixed views on targets and their implementation: assessments of the WCC initiative. As described in Chapter Three, this provided a framework for outcomes, governance and competencies relevant for commissioning but it was also a performance management process. Although originally a developmental process, WCC (Department of Health, 2007a) and its associated guidance and assurance framework was considered an influential performance management regime, although commissioning through partnerships was less well developed. WCC was seen as an important route for improving health outcomes and tackling health inequalities through encouraging a systematic approach to the commissioning cycle, knowledge management and prioritisation. In particular, it had increased the emphasis on performance management of health outcomes. Failure to meet minimum standards could result in further action being taken through SHAs and, in extreme cases, PCTs could be subject to a failure regime. Assessment of performance was likely to determine the degree of commissioning autonomy involved – an important incentive. Also, a league table of PCTs was published, which encouraged good practice and benchmarking of activities across commissioning organisations.

Interviewees from all case study sites considered WCC an effective assurance process allowing PCTs to benchmark their progress against best practice (although some sites considered that their health and wellbeing activities were well advanced already, with WCC making little difference). Interviewees in four sites felt that WCC had allowed the health and wellbeing agenda to be taken forward through a focus on health outcomes and a shift in power between commissioners and providers, giving commissioners more freedom to specify outcomes. In a discussion of smoking cessation services, one interviewee commented:

> 'What we'd be doing is saying well actually this is what the evidence tells us about effective smoking cessation, these are the sorts of levels of activity we want to see, these are the sorts of interventions we want to see, these are the sorts of places we want to see them, and the means by which

they're discharged, here's the deal, who wants to run this?'
(Director of strategy, site 7)

Some interviewees considered that the WCC cycle addressed some of
the weaknesses of process-driven performance management regimes.
For example, a focus on health outcomes and competencies two and
five in particular (working in partnership and assessing knowledge)
brought an increased emphasis on commissioning for health outcomes:

> 'There seems to be a policy shift as a result of world
> class commissioning that pushes us that way because we
> will be performance managed and therefore incentivised
> on performance in relation to life expectancy, health
> inequalities and the suite of public health outcome areas that
> we've determined as part of our world class commissioning
> approach.' (DPH, site 6)

At a local level, as shown in Chapter Two, there was often a deliberate
reshaping of organisational roles to reflect the governance arrangements
implied by WCC.

Lessons for performance management and public health

The experience with targets raises some generic issues for public
sector management. Smith (2013) outlines six key questions: (1) who
should choose the targets; (2) what targets should be chosen; (3) when
should outcomes be used as a basis for targets; (4) how should targets be
measured and set; (5) how should cross-ministerial targets be handled;
and (6) what accountability mechanisms should be attached to targets?

While the perverse consequences of a multitude of targets had
already been recognised by the Labour government and their numbers
somewhat reduced, the coalition government largely abandoned them,
replacing them with indicators and 'national ambitions'. Since 2010,
the emphasis has moved away from centrally imposed targets and
performance assessment frameworks to self-assessed outcomes through
the creation of outcomes frameworks for health, public health and
social care.

The joint strategic needs assessment (JSNA) guidance (Department
of Health, 2013a: 13) notes that:

> evidence based outcome measures ... can also be used by
> boards as a way of demonstrating progress in working
> together to improve health and care outcomes. However,
> they are not performance management tools, and are
> primarily designed to provide transparent measurement of
> progress, and focus the system on improving outcomes for
> everyone. Boards may also wish to consider developing local
> measures to demonstrate progress against their JSNAs and
> JHWSs [joint health and wellbeing strategies].

Improving life expectancy and addressing health inequalities became
an overarching outcome indicator for the public health outcomes
framework, but priorities are a matter for local authorities and decided
through mechanisms for local democratic accountability. In line with
this, information on key aspects, such as premature mortality by local
authority area and performance compared with similar areas, are
made available (Public Health England, 2013) and intended to inform
local debate. The framework has four domains: improving the wider
determinants of health; health protection; health improvement; and
healthcare public health and preventing premature mortality but they
are specifically not used for performance management.

As membership-based commissioning organisations, clinical
commissioning groups (CCGs) reflect greater professional accountability
for outcomes rather than accountability through the previous system
of centralised targets for PCTs, although they are accountable to NHS
England for certain indicators in the NHS Outcomes Framework.
There are also standards and statutory requirements in place, including
the NHS Constitution. The term 'targets' no longer appears but the
quality of health services commissioned by CCGs is described in NHS
England's 'outcomes indicator set', developed from the five domains
of the NHS Outcomes Framework. It is emphasised that this is a tool
for local priority setting rather a system of assessment or performance
management. Nevertheless, an assurance process is in place through
NHS England's local area teams (LATs) to demonstrate effective use of
public funds, although, just as was the case for WCC, the developmental
side of assurance is emphasised. CCGs, like PCTs before them, have
to produce an annual report. There are quarterly 'delivery dashboards',
annual assessments by the LATs and statutory powers of intervention if
assurance, development and support processes fail. They are, therefore,
increasingly beginning to resemble the former PCTs.

The outcomes frameworks provide benchmarking data and, while outcome measures are less liable to distortion, it is argued that some process measures can still provide a useful basis for targets (Smith, 2013).

With the relocation of public health responsibilities into local authorities, there is the possibility that public health priorities will continue to be displaced, although in this case by statutory requirements for local authority services rather than by the secondary care services. It is also possible that indicators in domains related to core local authority services will be prioritised over those areas previously prioritised by PCTs, namely healthcare public health and preventing premature mortality. Just as was the case for definitions of commissioning for health and wellbeing, summarised in Chapter Three, public health in local authorities can be considered as the sum total of what is already carried out. While the creation of a ring-fenced public health budget will help to ensure the provision of preventive services, there is considerable freedom in its use and it will not be ring-fenced over the longer term. It remains to be seen whether longer-term public health priorities will be neglected in the face of more pressing and immediate demands.

There remains some scepticism over the extent to which performance management can be substantially reduced, however. The Health Committee on commissioning noted, for example, that: 'We think that it is unrealistic to imagine that the NHS will be able to operate effectively without some means of performance management' (House of Commons Health Committee, 2011: para. 88). Targets are being continued in the context of CCG incentive arrangements, where payment of a quality premium for CCGs will be dependent on meeting targets including (a) maximum 18-week waits from referral to treatment; (b) maximum four-hour waits in Accident and Emergency departments; (c) maximum 62-day waits from urgent GP referral to first definitive treatment for cancer; and (d) maximum 8-minute responses for Category A (Red 1) ambulance calls (NHS England, 2013). The history of CCGs to date has been one of increasing development of assurance processes.

The importance of ownership of a public health agenda across a local authority area was emphasised in the case study sites, and the subsequent transfer of public health to local authorities has been generally welcomed. While local authority responsibility for public health is expected to promote local responsiveness and capacity to influence social determinants of health and health equity within a context of democratic accountability, the accountability arrangements and effectiveness of new HWBs are yet to be tested. As noted in the report from the House of Commons Communities and Local Government Committee on public health in local authorities (2013), accountability remains unclear and HWBs, although statutory organisations, lack funds or formal powers and will therefore need to influence through partnerships.

Finally there is the issue of the assurance framework associated with WCC. Many saw this as a process that affirmed the importance of a public health approach, with its starting point in the process of health needs assessment and its emphasis on mandatory outcomes of improving health and addressing health inequalities. Many of its features remain, such as the JSNA. However, responsibility for a public health-led commissioning cycle has become dispersed. The findings of the study suggest there would be benefits in developing a more systematic and integrated approach to commissioning health improvement, health care and social care services across a local authority area, building on the WCC model, but in a new context. It remains to be seen how far HWBs will be able to fulfil this role.

Conclusions

Before the introduction of WCC in 2007, the *Commissioning framework for health and well-being* (Department of Health, 2007a) noted that incentives did not yet 'fully support the delivery of better health and well-being', that skills for forward-looking commissioning and focusing on prevention were scarce, and that health and local authorities were 'structurally complex and culturally different organisations' (para. 1.12). At a local level, there was evidence from the study that the complex system of targets and regulation which framed priority setting within commissioning organisations imperfectly translated government intentions for promoting health and wellbeing. Problems of complexity, lack of alignment of targets across agencies, an emphasis on short-term process variables and an unspoken hierarchy of targets combined to ensure that an emphasis on health and wellbeing largely existed in spite of, rather than as a result of, performance management frameworks. Intentions to streamline targets were not successful and often added to the target burden. While targets cross-cut and were interrelated, different layers and separate performance management arrangements, combined with the sheer numbers of targets, created difficulties for commissioners. The targets related to improving health and addressing health inequalities had to take their place among numerous competing targets, only some of which were prioritised in practice. As other studies have shown (Lipsky, 1980), there is a great deal of variation in implementation and there is little evidence that governance arrangements can be the sole driver of performance (Davies et al., 2005: 76). Nevertheless, there was a wide recognition that the existence of targets focused attention and shaped prioritisation, and that there was concerted attention at a policy level. Bevan and Hood (2006) demonstrated improvement in key NHS priorities, such as hospital waiting times, although this was also associated with a wide range of gaming responses (such as ambulances waiting outside hospitals until patients could be seen within the four-hour target) which distorted the data. They argued that 'nobody would want to return to the NHS performance before the introduction of targets' (2006: 421). Gaming strategies were not necessarily interpreted as an argument against targets as part of performance management but as an incentive for modifying targets to make them less vulnerable to gaming and to maximise their social benefits. Nevertheless, the system for WCC was seen by some interviewees as a counterbalance, combining an outcomes-based approach with a systematic process, underpinned by commissioning competencies.

Whatever the governance arrangements in force, this analysis raises a number of generic questions for a public health agenda. To what extent do governance arrangements prioritise a public health agenda and, even if they are intended to do so, does this occur in practice or do more immediate short-term demands displace a longer-term perspective on public health risks? A multiplicity of targets almost inevitably leads to a hierarchy of targets, and lack of alignment in performance management at a national level is likely to be replicated at the level of local organisations. PCT 'core business' – that is, the quality of health care services – dominated, with public health sometimes described as an 'earned agenda' subject to savings having been made in other areas or viable only in the context of growth money. It was clear that many of the sources of ill health lay outside the control of PCTs and it was therefore difficult to hold them to account for a failure to narrow the health inequalities gap. It remains the case that focusing on the role of local organisations in addressing health inequalities – whether the former PCTs, as in the study, or local authorities with their public health responsibilities – may serve to distract attention from wider changes required across government if substantial improvements are to be achieved.

Notes

[1] See: www.publicservices.ac.uk/.

[2] See: www.nice.org.uk/localgovernment/PublicHealthBriefingsForLocal Government.jsp.

CHAPTER FIVE

Levers for change (2): incentives

This chapter focuses on the use of financial incentives and contractual flexibilities for encouraging the provision and uptake of preventive services. It has been argued in the context of health care systems that the use of incentives reflects a shift from 'command and control' regulation towards the encouragement of entrepreneurial behaviour (Saltman, 2002). While the relationships between governance and incentives are not straightforward and outcomes cannot be predicted from particular modes of governance (Davies et al., 2005), governance through markets, for example, will encourage the deployment of performance-linked incentives agreed through a contractual route. The increased emphasis on the use of incentives over the period of the study was consistent with the introduction of market-based reforms in health care which emphasised choice and competition as routes for improving quality and involved the separation of commissioning from the provision of services.

While the use of financial incentives in health care has become increasingly influential (Mannion and Davies, 2008), there are many different kinds of incentives. As illustrated in the previous chapter, governance arrangements, such as performance management regimes, can themselves exert powerful incentive effects. It was argued, for example (Department of Health, 2007a: 50), that 'greater alignment of accountability mechanisms should form an important part of an incentive framework, creating both greater transparency and strong drivers to collaborate'. Incentives can span intrinsic satisfaction and external rewards, including, but not limited to financial rewards, and can be used to discourage or encourage. Whether directed at individuals, groups or organisations, incentives are considered an important lever for achieving change and there are many possible routes through which commissioners can incentivise providers (across the NHS, the private sector or the voluntary and community sector [VCS]) to improve their performance or to provide additional services. Commissioners can also incentivise individuals to change their lifestyles or access specific services.

The chapter begins by reviewing financial and other incentives, locates debates on incentives in a theoretical framework and considers some of the characteristics of 'incentive contracts', before summarising the range of incentives available to commissioners at the time of the study and views of their impact. There follows a discussion of local enhanced services (LES), the most popular route for incentivising public health services at the time, with the aim of illustrating benefits and drawbacks of incentivising preventive services.

Incentives in context

The use of financial incentives in health care, including preventive care, has been subject to extensive critical assessment (Kane et al., 2004; Davies et al., 2005). A review of the links between financial incentives, health care providers and quality improvement (Christianson et al., 2009) demonstrated that financial incentives were ineffective in improving quality, when used in isolation. A systematic review of pay-for-performance (P4P) schemes, many of which covered preventive services, found mixed evidence that such schemes improved quality of care. The review highlighted shortcomings in the current evidence base, which was unable to address key questions such as the optimal duration for payments or whether effects endured after rewards were removed (Petersen et al., 2006). A study of P4P schemes in Massachusetts, USA, which also covered preventive services such as those for children and adolescents, found no evidence of positive effects on the quality of care (Pearson et al., 2008). Taking a broader perspective, McDonald et al. (2013) draw attention to the shortcomings of locally developed schemes, emphasising that technical aspects, such as developing indicators, setting thresholds and identifying rewards need expert input.

Research has also shown some benefits of incentives built into the Quality and Outcomes Framework (QOF), the voluntary P4P element of the general medical services (GMS) contract. Millett et al. (2007) concluded that financial incentives introduced in primary care increased smoking cessation advice given by primary care staff and reduced the percentage of people with diabetes who smoked, with improvements generally greatest in the groups with the poorest performance before these incentives were introduced. McDonald et al. (2010) showed that incentives modify primary care professionals' behaviour, reducing variation in the quality of care, and contribute to meeting targets, while McDonald et al. (2008) showed that local contextual factors may influence the impact of national incentive schemes. The former GP fundholding scheme also demonstrated the responsiveness of GPs to financial incentives (Gosden and Torgerson, 1997). However, a study of the impact of the QOF on health inequalities (Dixon et al., 2010) showed limited impact and suggested that changes in the current incentive structure were needed – a conclusion also reached in a study which showed that financial incentives in the QOF were not designed to maximise health gain (Fleetcroft et al., 2012). These studies tend to confirm Mannion and Davies' (2008) view that the use of incentives in health care lacks a coherent theory with predictive validity. What kinds of incentives are most effective (and in which contexts), and the levels, frequency and duration of the incentives required, remain relevant and largely unanswered questions for commissioners. Other relevant questions include safety (for example, risks of unintended consequences) and 'efficiency' or budgetary impact (Leary and Palmer, 2009).

However, incentives take many different forms other than the financial incentives (such as performance-related pay) with which they are most often associated. Their use needs to be considered in the light of other sources of motivation, arising from different organisational contexts and cultures as well as individual motivational factors. These include, among others, a shared culture and purpose (Mannion et al., 2003) as reflected in a public service ethos, for example; performance-related freedoms; positive feedback; peer review; and the use of benchmarking as a route for critically assessing performance against relevant comparators.

The wide range of possible motivational factors (and the complex relationships between them) underlines the importance of drawing on social, organisational and behavioural studies in order to understand influences on performance. The use of financial incentives, for example, may lead to a reduction in intrinsic motivation and interest, or a reduced sense of competence (McDonald et al., 2008). Davies et al. (2005:7) point out that recent studies in political science, public administration and policy analysis 'take issue with the language of incentives and stress the importance of building solidarity and acknowledging commitment, especially in "joined up" community governance contexts'. They argue that building individualised incentives into the ways that organisations are designed risks 'dismantling notions of the public good'. On a similar theme, Newman (2001, quoted in Davies et al., 2005), distinguishes between 'solidaristic incentives' reflected in self and in network governance and 'individualised' incentives reflected in hierarchies and market governance. These distinctions raise questions over the balance of individualised and 'solidaristic incentives' across a system and the likely impact.

In addition, the impact of incentives can be unpredictable where the system as a whole is taken into account. Systems can incorporate conflicting incentives (as in the NHS in England, where there are incentives for primary care to manage demand and for NHS Trusts to increase acute sector activity). Solidaristic incentives (through partnerships, for example) may be encouraged at the same time as the search for competitive advantage; and incentives may be differently applied across different levels of governance. Incentives can have the potential for coercion (Pearson and Lieber, 2009) and have implications for autonomy (Le Grand et al., 2009). They therefore need to be considered on ethical grounds as well as in relation to their cost-effectiveness or feasibility.

Given the range of individual, organisational and system-level incentives that may be in place, reflecting the interests of multiple stakeholders, there is continued debate over the extent to which different kinds or permutations of incentives cohere, conflict or result in perverse and unintended consequences. In a qualitative study on the views of managers on the pattern of incentives and regulatory structures in relation to promoting health, Hunter and Marks (2005) argued that the fact that public health was largely considered as part of the NHS rather than as part of a wider health public health system lay behind the ways in which incentives and performance management regimes had been skewed towards health care. Important themes to consider, therefore, are the relative importance of financial as opposed to other incentives and the potential for incentives in one part of a health system to have unforeseen or undesirable consequences in another.

Theoretical approaches

Many disciplines contribute to an understanding of incentives and of their influence on decision making and behaviour change. A review by Davies et al. (2005) assessed the contribution of various disciplines, including economics, organisational theory, political theory and psychology, to understanding links between governance and outcomes through incentive effects. They noted that economics as a discipline lends particular weight to the use of incentives. However, understanding the different heuristics underlying intuitive judgement has become increasingly influential, as has 'nudge' economics, in influencing behaviour change (Thaler and Sunstein, 2008). For example, responses may depend on the method used to elicit them (the anchoring heuristic), while 'nudge' economics explores how the 'choice environment' can be designed to encourage (or 'nudge') individuals to make beneficial choices. The tendency towards 'doing nothing' (Thaler and Sunstein, 2008) means that if individuals are offered a choice with a default option, many will 'choose' this option. Well-designed default rules can act as powerful nudges to encourage particular choices. This has been used in policies to encourage organ donation, as in the decision taken by the Welsh Assembly in 2013, where if no action has been taken to opt out of organ donation this is taken to imply consent. The tendency not to act is particularly marked when benefits and costs are separated in time: this can apply, for example, to failure to 'invest in health'. Policies need to recognise and address this imbalance either by increasing present benefits or decreasing present costs and providing feedback mechanisms to narrow perceptions of the gap between benefits and costs.

In order to provide a theoretical context for understanding financial and other incentives and, in particular, the use of incentive contracts, the following section summarises how incentives might work – through markets, decision-making heuristics and contracts. This builds on part of a review by Davies et al. (2005), which used a Governance Incentives–Outcomes (GIO) model to analyse incentives and outcomes associated with governance modes, including markets, hierarchies and networks. As background to the study findings, four theoretical economic approaches are summarised: neoclassical economics; game theory; institutional economics; and experimental economics (Box 5.1). The different theoretical approaches underline the complexity of designing effective incentives, as the design needs to take account of factors influencing individual decision making ('heuristics' and the 'choice environment'); the potential for incentives to result in gaming strategies; and the interplay of incentives at different levels of decision making across a whole system, which is hard to predict. The study was mainly concerned with system-level incentives and how commissioners used incentives and contractual flexibilities in their commissioning decisions. These are discussed in the next section.

Box 5.1: Theoretical approaches to incentives

Neoclassical economics, the foundation of most economic theory, is concerned with the working of the market, how organisations function under different market structures, why markets fail and the interventions that arise as a result of lack of market 'equilibrium'. These interventions can include national targets, regulation and taxes. Health care does not fulfil the conditions for market equilibrium: for example, there are monopolistic organisations and unequal access to and use of, information. In markets, incentives are an inbuilt part of the price system, working to match supply and demand. The premises of neoclassical economics have been widely criticised, in particular in respect of 'scientism' in relation to the 'market', as inappropriate for a social phenomenon, and assumptions of rationality (the latter being increasingly addressed through game theory and experimental economics, below).

Game theory is concerned with the complexity of interactive decision making, the potential for opportunism and the unintended consequences that may arise from using various incentive structures. It deals with concepts of uncertainty, risk and 'principal–agent' problems using mathematical models. Principal–agent theory provides one focus for research on incentives, where the principal's responsibility is to manipulate incentives to achieve the best possible results from the agent. It considers differences in information and motivation between 'principals' and 'agents' and outcomes of rational individual decisions taken under uncertainty which gives rise to 'gaming' by individuals as they interact during the decision-making process. This can result in 'opportunism', that is, efforts to realise individual gains through a lack of honesty in transactions (Williamson, 1973). There are differences in the extent of information held between agents: employers may not know how much effort employees are making, particularly where outputs are difficult to measure. These difficulties explain why commissioners use incentives, contracts and performance indicators to manage providers, but the unintended consequences of these approaches should also be considered. While neoclassical theory assumes that people will only do what they perceive to be in their own interests, game theory recognises that individuals are likely to be a combination of 'knights and knaves' (Le Grand, 2003) that is, motivated both by self-interest and altruism, and may also value non-pecuniary gains such as fair treatment of themselves and others (Williamson, 1973). These different motivations therefore need to be reflected in policy reforms and Davies and colleagues (2005) note that game theory is being developed to tackle some of the complexities of decision making in the public sector.

Institutional economics draws on elements of game theory and is concerned with understanding the 'science' of contracts and the use of incentives within contracts. In this context, contracts are defined as a way of mediating the relationship between commissioners (principals) and providers (agents) and theories are based on an analysis of principal–agent relationships in hierarchical and market–type arrangements. Institutional economics also sheds light on contractual relationships, defining the associated costs as 'transaction costs' (Marini and Street, 2007). Incentive contracts are one way of ensuring that the 'agent' bears some of the risk or responsibility for the outcomes of their actions. There are several principles governing the design of optimal incentive contracts and these can all be applied by commissioners (Milgrom and Roberts 1992: 240–1; Williamson, 1973). Conversely, if such principles are not applied, incentives may fail to achieve their intended effect, as discussed with reference to the study. However, if outcomes are difficult to measure, then optimal incentive schemes are difficult to develop and implement (Davies et al., 2005).

Experimental economics draws on psychological theories, focusing on how decisions are made in practice. It can, therefore, help to understand the impact of different incentives on decision making, including behaviour change. As tasks become more complex, individuals may adopt simplifying decision-making strategies. This means that decisions may be biased in systematic ways, notwithstanding high stakes or financial rewards being made available (Thaler, 1994). Tversky and Kahneman (1974) originally proposed three heuristics underlying intuitive judgement but which can lead to predictable, systematic errors. Experiments support the view that individuals tend to give too little weight to prior information and too much weight to new information (Thaler, 1994: 154). Many other heuristics have been developed. For example, prospect theory (Kahneman and Tversky, 1979) has demonstrated, through experiment, that people's attitudes to risks over gains may differ from their attitudes toward risks over losses, and that outcomes with certainty are over-weighted relative to uncertain outcomes. In addition to biases associated with heuristics, other systematic errors can occur during decision making, such as the 'sunk costs' effect, where judgement may be based on costs already incurred. For example, if a fixed payment has to be made for weight management classes, participants may be more likely to attend than if they just pay for each class attended (Thaler, 1994: 193).

Source: Adapted from Marks et al., 2011a.

Commissioners' use of incentives

In specifying contracts, commissioners can include financial incentives aligned to their commissioning priorities in order, for example, to encourage a range of providers to improve their performance, increase choice, meet specific targets or provide additional services. As described in Chapter Two, the NHS in England has been characterised as a 'quasi-market', combining a public sector organisation with market features. The framework for world class commissioning (WCC), for example, explicitly required commissioners to 'effectively stimulate the market to meet demand and secure required clinical and health and wellbeing outcomes' (Department of Health, 2007c: 18–19). The controversial 'section 75' of the Health and Social Care Act 2012 cemented requirements to procure NHS services in England through competitive tendering. In relation to public health services, local authorities are encouraged to 'contract for services with a wide range of providers across the public, private and voluntary sectors and to incentivise and reward those organisations to deliver the best outcomes for their population' (Secretary of State for Health, 2010b: para. 4.23). This can include 'grant funding' for local communities to 'take ownership of some highly focused preventive activities, such as volunteering, peer support, befriending and social networks'.

The creation of 'optimal incentive contracts' by commissioners is complex and four principles have been developed to encourage effective use of incentives (Milgrom and Roberts, 1992: 240–1). First is the 'informativeness principle', which means that performance measures should effectively measure effort and exclude factors outside the agents' control. This often involves collecting activity data related to the incentive. Second is the 'incentive intensity' principle, which concerns the optimal level of the incentive in relation to factors such as marginal returns, precision of measurement, levels of risk and responsiveness to the incentive. Third is the 'monitoring intensity' principle, which implies that more resources should be spent monitoring when it is desirable to give strong incentives, for example, if there is substantial variation in performance or performance is uniformly poor. Finally the 'equal compensation principle' means that incentives should ensure that the marginal returns earned by the agent are equal for all tasks the agent undertakes. Providing strong incentives for only some activities can cause agents to reduce effort in others.

The study provided examples of how each of these principles were (or were not) reflected in incentive contracts for preventive services, illustrating broader issues over the impact of individual and system incentives.

Incentives are not limited to professional or provider behaviour but may also be targeted at certain groups or individuals in order to encourage changes in lifestyle or to improve the take up of services (Le Grand et al., 2009). For example, some primary care trusts (PCTs) in the study had begun to offer incentives for lifestyle change, sometimes in areas where PCTs needed to meet targets. Incentives included the use of loyalty cards with points added for healthy behaviours, which could be converted to benefits through a local social enterprise, and cinema tickets to promote participation in outreach screening programmes for Chlamydia. Whether these approaches proved an efficient method of targeting those most at risk remained unclear. There is a growing body of evidence that financial incentives targeted at individuals can lead to changes in short-term behaviour – such as smoking cessation, physical activity or weight loss – but it is less clear that changes persist after financial rewards have ceased (Le Grand et al., 2009). This view was reflected by interviewees in the study, who considered that incentives were more effective for encouraging uptake of screening services, than for long-term behaviour change. Commissioners of health improvement services will therefore need to be aware of the impact of individual-level incentives on encouraging healthy behaviour, taking account of the extent to which changes are sustained (Kane et al., 2004; Oliver, 2009).

At national level, rewards may be offered for meeting national targets or achieving improvement. As one example, the public health White Paper, *Healthy lives, healthy people* (Secretary of State for Health, 2010b; Department of Health, 2011b) introduced a 'Health Premium' (from 2015–16), a cash incentive for local authorities making good progress on public health indicators drawn from the public health outcomes framework. However, demonstrating the dangers of considering incentives in isolation, this proposal proved controversial and it was argued that the incentive had the potential for perverse consequences, that is, increasing inequalities rather than helping to reduce them and rewarding richer areas at the expense of poorer ones (House of Commons Communities and Local Government Committee, 2013). Moreover, if health outcomes improved, core allocations would be reduced. The time lag between interventions and changes in health outcomes and the impact of population churn were further complications.

The following section is limited to the options available to commissioners at the time of the study and explores in detail the extent to which LESs, reward schemes and contractual flexibilities were effectively deployed for promoting health and wellbeing. It draws both on interviews carried out in the 10 case study sites and on the national survey.

The range of available incentives

At the time of the study, a range of incentives related to activity, performance, partnership and quality improvement were in place and these are discussed in turn. Most were included in contracts and delivery plans but some, such as Spearhead status funding and rewards for practice-based commissioners, fell outside a contractual framework. Rewards for practice-based commissioning (PBC) and for incentives for preventive services are discussed in more detail in subsequent sections.

System incentives in opposition: payment by results

Payment by results (PbR), phased in from 2003/4 for the NHS in England, meant that hospitals were reimbursed for activity, using a fixed tariff which reflected the national average. It was seen as a lever to reduce costs, introducing an incentive for hospital trusts to compete for patients and making it theoretically possible for commissioners to choose between providers. Linked to activity (rather than the results implied in the title), PbR has steadily replaced the previous system of block contracting with providers (Marini and Street, 2007). By 2008/9, it covered 45% of all secondary health care purchased by PCTs and has since risen to about 60% of average hospital activity (Appleby et al., 2012). PbR is intended to improve efficiency and support patient choice, but has also been criticised for rewarding increased activity in the acute sector, rather than reducing demand through community-based schemes, coordination of care or preventive initiatives.

While relevant for certain aspects of secondary care, this payment system nevertheless reflects an inbuilt system incentive that not only worked against a focus on prevention but also against a coordinated and system-wide approach to demand management. In this sense, it reflected a lack of coherence across the reform programme as a whole, in that the emphasis on prevention was not reflected in the payment systems for acute care. This view was reiterated by interviewees in the study:

> 'The difficulty can be countering the perverse incentives in the system, and one of the biggest ones of those is payment by results, period. It's just, in terms of commissioning for health and wellbeing, payment by results is almost a disaster, because it's not payment by results at all, it's payment by activity. And if you just think about it with the pure accountancy hat on from a hospital point of view, if they're paid for admissions, then there's no incentive to reduce admissions.' (Director of strategy, site 3)

PbR was not the only example. Monitor, the independent regulator for NHS Foundation Trusts (set up in 2004) required trusts to make a surplus, as one interviewee commented:

> 'At the other end of the spectrum you've got Foundation Trusts who as a requirement of their operating licence with Monitor, requires them to produce a surplus. So they have no incentive to do other than to suck more and more work into their hospital or whatever their institution is. Now there is a complete absence of any notion that these things are aligned.' (Director of strategy, site 7)

As mentioned earlier, the impact of individual incentives was reduced if incentives in the system conflicted or were misaligned. The consensus was that PbR worked against commissioning for health and wellbeing and it was difficult, despite demand management initiatives, to release resources from acute care to reinvest in preventive services. In the same way, demand management initiatives in primary care could lead to tensions with secondary care. One interviewee identified tensions between PbR and PBC as follows:

'Payment by results and practice-based commissioning, if working effectively, are going to divide primary and secondary care working effectively together, and we need to work out very carefully how to not let that happen locally.' (PEC chair, site 5)

Evaluations suggest that PbR was considered to have 'sharpened incentives and introduced greater clarity into the contracting process' (Mannion et al., 2008: 82), leading to modest increases in activity with little or no detrimental impact on quality (Farrar et al., 2007; Audit Commission, 2009b). While PbR has lowered the costs of price negotiation, costs associated with volume control, data collection, contract monitoring and contract enforcement are higher (Marini and Street, 2007). These changes in transaction costs affect both providers and commissioners. It has been argued that the system of PbR is more suited to elective care and less suited to services where competition and choice are limited (Appleby et al., 2012) and that it is only one of a range of possible policy instruments, including a wider range of payment systems.

Preventive services fell outside the scope of PbR (Department of Health, 2007e). However, there were a few examples of tariffs being included in contracts to reflect health improvement targets. Around 14% of PCTs responding to the national survey were using tariffs for preventive services, mostly for smoking cessation, and an example of mandatory tariffs for health improvement services is provided in Box 5.2. One of the focus groups conducted as part of the study discussed tariffs for health improvement services with one participant noting:

'But if you think about smoking cessation services, weight management services, these are health wellness services, is what I call them, and if you have a tariff concept in wellness services, you'd actually really focus people's attention on delivering it cost-effectively, commissioning it cost-effectively, and I think it changes behaviour. So I think there are some policy incentives, if you like, that we really haven't explored fully in public health terms.' (National focus group)

The tariff could be weighted towards underserved populations with the aim of actively encouraging effective targeting. There is, therefore, scope for better specification of contracts for preventive services.

Box 5.2: Tariffs for lifestyle risk management services

The former West Midlands Strategic Health Authority introduced mandatory tariffs for lifestyle risk management services such as health trainers, smoking cessation clinics, and expert patient programmes (Wyatt, 2008). The aim was to address supply-side barriers by providing financial incentives to expand the provision of preventive services. Providers accredited by a PCT were free to recruit participants and provide services in line with a detailed service specification. Providers also had to provide activity information for audit purposes. Tariffs were payable for achievement of specific outcomes, or intermediate outcomes, rather than for activity. Payments were adjusted to reflect the effort required to recruit specific groups, and to discourage adverse selection, or 'cherry picking'. There were also higher payments for pregnant women who stopped smoking. Transition payments were available (to reduce the risk of short-term financial instability), and auditable codes of conduct were written into contracts (to discourage gaming and to help align principal-agent incentives).

Source: Adapted from Marks et al., 2011a.

Incentive contracts: commissioning for quality and innovation

High quality care for all, the final report of the NHS Next Stage Review by Lord Darzi (Secretary of State for Health, 2008), emphasised better use of a range of incentives, along with improved information and data on effectiveness, as key routes for driving up quality. One of the new financial incentives proposed was 'commissioning for quality and innovation' (CQUIN), where a small percentage of hospital income depended on attaining certain outcomes. It was introduced in the NHS Operating Framework for 2009/10 (Department of Health, 2008c) with the intention of linking payment to quality improvement in 2009/10 contracts.

PCT interviewees discussed the idea of commissioning for quality through CQUIN, but this was considered only in respect of acute and mental health service providers. However, in discussion, the complexity of introducing such payments emerged, reflecting difficulties in implementing optimal incentive contracts in relation to the 'monitoring intensity' and 'incentive intensity' principles discussed earlier. A director of strategy noted:

> 'Actually it wasn't always straightforward to think what those quality indicators could be. It was really easy to think of what the topic matters were, you know, there are things that are very important to us, but actually nailing them down to something that (a) can be measured, (b) can be measured without too much added grief, (c) where there wasn't a get out of jail free card for the provider in the sense that oh well, you know, actually we didn't perform well but actually that wasn't our fault, that was somebody else's fault, you know, you could be specific about what the provider's role was in that part of the quality measure, and then setting a realistic target for the improvement of the quality, is actually really difficult.' (Director of strategy, site 3)

CQUIN was generally focused on better health outcomes for patients, and not on a preventive agenda, although there was evidence of using CQUIN (or quality indicators which pre-dated its introduction in acute contracts) to promote preventive services. There were examples of incentivising smoking cessation services (for maternity services), screening all elective patients for smoking status and for encouraging Accident and Emergency Departments to share information on alcohol-related injuries with other agencies. However, it was pointed out that these targets were difficult to monitor and it was possible that some interventions, such as smoking cessation, could be better located in primary care.

There were four national CQUIN goals for 2013/14 and additional local goals are subject to local agreement between commissioners and providers (NHS Commissioning Board, 2013). Providers are paid only if the goals are reached and these goals have to reflect improvements beyond those expected as standard.

Pay for performance: the Quality and Outcomes Framework

The QOF was first introduced in 2004 as part of the new contract, and is regularly revised. It was designed to reward quality in primary care based on evidence-based process indicators across four domains, and includes several preventive indicators. It is an ambitious P4P scheme and as such, reflects a move 'away from placing implicit trust in individuals and organisations to carry out their duties, towards actively managing their performance' (McDonald et al., 2010: 9). Local extensions to the nationally agreed contract were made available in some PCTs through 'QOF plus' schemes, often designed to address QOF weaknesses related to preventive activities. However, standard QOF payments form part of a national contract and are nationally negotiated. They are not, therefore, open to commissioner influence. The QOF is revised annually and the 2013/14 QOF includes a new public health domain to reflect commitments in the public health White Paper (Secretary of State for Health, 2010b) that the QOF should include evidence-based public health and primary prevention indicators. These include lifestyle advice for patients with hypertension, blood pressure monitoring, smoking cessation support and screening services (NHS Employers, 2013).

The QOF focuses on 'activity' and workload and provides little information on outcomes, a point reiterated in the report of the House of Commons Health Committee on health inequalities (House of Commons Health Committee 2009: 9) in the context of the importance of measuring the number of successful smoking quitters rather than numbers simply given advice. There is a lack of baseline measurement for the framework and it is therefore impossible to know if real changes are being measured or current practice is simply being described (Wanless et al., 2007), although it seems clear that it has led to improvements in recording practice activities.

The QOF has also been criticised for its lack of capacity to incentivise a population-based approach to health and wellbeing. There is little incentive to proactively identify populations at risk not currently on disease registers, a task which is key to targeting populations most at risk of premature mortality. This is being addressed, in part, through rolling out the NHS Health Check programme, the responsibility of local authorities since 2013, and likely to involve a range of providers.

There was frustration among some interviewees over the inflexibility and limited opportunities for performance managing national GMS contracts, despite initiatives such as 'balanced scorecards' (combining quality and efficiency indicators) or monitoring QOF points:

> 'The general medical contract for GPs needs to be taken apart root and branch and put back together again on evidence- and policy-based medicine. That won't happen because there are too many vested interests.... But if it did happen, you could theoretically transform the landscape by making it much more cost efficient and much more effective in terms of curative service, rehabilitative services and preventative services. All the rest is flittering around

by seizing on levers that don't actually work, in my view, because they're too complex.' (DPH, site 1)

Some interviewees considered that the QOF had encouraged proactive case finding but most interviewees considered that, as currently configured, it did not adequately incentivise a proactive and population-based approach to health and wellbeing services. PCTs therefore experienced difficulties in securing change where there was no financial reward.

'We have the situation where because of the central contract for GPs, I have GPs saying it's not my job to reduce blood pressure or BMI [body mass index], cholesterol. I'm not paid to manage risk; I'm paid to manage the consequence of risk. If you want me to change people's lifestyle then pay me to do that.' (NED [non-executive director], site 7)

The QOF was also more likely to act as an incentive for smaller practices. If the QOF was to support improved health and wellbeing, new QOF points were needed:

'I think the government needs to put its money where its mouth is and it needs to change some of the QOF points to say we want a really assertive approach to obesity, we want a really assertive approach to — particularly with parents that have got children because this thing is in the families — to smoking, to drinking, to drug taking, to exercise.' (PCT chair, site 3)

In response to some of these shortcomings, in the first phase of the study, two PCTs planned to develop 'QOF Plus' schemes to build in extra health and wellbeing indicators and provide additional rewards to high-performing practices, while offering incentives for improvement for poorer-performing practices. In the national survey, PCT respondents were asked whether they had plans to extend QOF to incentivise health and wellbeing and just 16 PCTs claimed to have plans. In terms of how this group described how QOF would be extended, the following areas were cited: smoking cessation, cardiovascular disease, obesity and diabetes.

While evaluations of the QOF suggest that it has the potential to narrow health inequalities (Doran et al., 2008) rates of exception reporting — where patients can be excluded from the calculation of performance – need to be taken into account when determining the actual impact (Sigfrid et al., 2006). However, as maximum payments for many indicators are made when 90% of eligible patients are treated, there is little financial incentive for GPs to offer services to those patients who arguably have the greatest capacity to benefit. A systematic review of the impact of the QOF on health outcomes and on non-incentivised services (Langdown and Peckham, 2013) demonstrated an improvement in some health outcomes, but a plateau was reached after a few years and measurement of outcome was, in any event, extremely limited and only one indicator – seizure-free epilepsy patients – reflected a health outcome. An illustration of 'the equal compensation principle', described earlier, is found in research evaluating the impact of the QOF in primary care on targeted and untargeted clinical practice. Campbell et al. (2009) showed, for example, that delivery of services rewarded with performance payments improved while untargeted services declined. Once targets were met, improvements in the quality of care slowed. Langdown and Peckham (2013) also showed a decline over the longer term in non-incentivised activities. As the QOF was originally developed as a payment tool, rather than a route for population health gain, this may account for some of its shortcomings from this perspective.

Taking a rather different approach, Bernstein et al. (2010) argued that reductions in NHS spending due to GPs 'assertively' addressing lifestyle risk factors such as smoking, obesity and alcohol consumption should be passed on in the form of larger PBC budgets, which would act as an incentive to improve preventive care. Unlike PBC, clinical commissioning groups (CCGs) are statutory budget holders and can aim to rebalance their investment. However, preventive services are now commissioned by local authorities: negotiation and coordination will therefore be required.

The 2004 GMS contract also opened up a range of commissioning flexibilities, including a system of direct and local enhanced services, and the ability to commission through alternative provider medical services (APMS). Other financial incentives fall outside a contractual framework. This applied to Spearhead status and rewards to practice-based commissioners. These are discussed in turn.

Incentives for partnership working: local area agreements

As discussed in Chapter Four, local area agreements (LAAs) were jointly agreed delivery plans for achieving the aims of the sustainable community strategy and were considered important for promoting a health and wellbeing agenda and partnership working. Rewards were available (through pump priming and a performance reward grant for achievement of 'stretch' targets). The reward was shared by all partners involved thus encouraging the pooling of budgets across a local authority area. However, it was argued (Gash et al., 2008) that financial incentives were small in relation to the administrative input involved.

Incentives through additional baseline funding: Spearhead status

The funding formula for PCTs included a health inequalities element and Spearhead areas had more to spend than the England average (Audit Commission, 2010). The Labour government ascribed Spearhead status to the fifth most deprived local authority areas in England and 88 PCTs (covering 70 local authorities) were designated as Spearhead areas in 2004 on the basis of data on deprivation, life expectancy, and mortality from cancer and heart disease. (In 2006, this was reduced to 62 PCTs, due to clustering.) Narrowing the life expectancy gap between the Spearhead areas and the rest of the country formed the basis of one of the national health inequalities targets. Half the sites in the study were Spearhead PCTs or contained Spearhead areas. Although associated with additional funding, the impact of Spearhead status was not extensive. A small number of PCT interviewees felt Spearhead status had raised their PCT's profile and increased the focus on public health and inequalities, including at board level, but most interviewees agreed that the impact was minimal:

> 'The impact, I'm not sure it's had any impact whatsoever. Well the point is do you need to be a Spearhead to know that you've got to get to grips with health and wellbeing and prevention. You're just going to do it anyway ... if you said is our work around health and wellbeing and prevention delivered because of being a Spearhead, no, it would have been done anyway.' (Director of commissioning, site 8)

While the extra funding associated with Spearhead status was acknowledged, none of the interviewees could give examples of how such funds had been spent to reduce inequalities or any Spearhead funded projects which had then been mainstreamed. It had simply formed part of the baseline:

> 'I'm sure any Spearhead money that ever did come through
> – again I wasn't here – has disappeared. We certainly haven't

> got any earmarked funds, I'm not aware of anything that
> says 'Spearhead money' here.' (DPH, site 8)

Two PCT interviewees felt there was a lack of accountability for the
performance of Spearhead areas:

> 'I certainly don't feel that anybody at the SHA [strategic
> health authority] has ever been held to account, in any way,
> shape or form, for the Spearhead area making different
> progress.' (Chief executive, site 2)

In order to put these findings in a national context, the national survey
questioned whether having Spearhead status acted as an incentive to
focus on health and wellbeing. Over half the respondents considered
there was little or no effect.

These results demonstrate that the lack of a contractual element or
of routine performance monitoring meant that this directed financial
payment was considered part of the baseline budget and was not
specifically targeted at inequalities in health.

Rewards for involvement in practice-based commissioning

Prior to the development of CCGs, many attempts had been made
to involve GPs in commissioning, including the total purchasing and
fundholding initiatives of the 1990s. At the time of the study, PBC
was the route through which GP practices engaged with PCTs in
commissioning, including activities such as reducing demand for acute
services through redesigning pathways of care. Clinical engagement
in commissioning activities had proved difficult to achieve and
difficulties in implementing PBC have been reviewed elsewhere
(Curry et al., 2008). Various incentives were put in place by PCTs to
encourage practice-based commissioners to engage in commissioning
and in designing services. However, once CCGs were established as
statutory commissioning organisations with their own budgets, service
redesign was largely incentivised through needing to achieve financial
sustainability. However, some of the tensions that have since emerged
in CCGs were prefigured in the study.

PBC was encouraged through payment of GPs for getting involved
(often through a PBC LES) and through their being able to use 70% of
any savings (freed-up resources [FUR]), derived from PBC initiatives
to reconfigure care or generate efficiency savings. There were also
other local approaches, such as innovation budgets, which provided

funds for developing and piloting ideas, or using half of any savings for developing pooled bids. This was seen as an incentive for partnership working and occurred in a case study site which had strong clinical leadership and collaboration with general practices.

A PBC LES could encourage monitoring of non-elective activity, public involvement in commissioning and management of budgets and, for FUR, it was clarified (Department of Health, 2007a: 51) that NHS funding could be used for a wide range of innovative measures to avoid hospital admission, including social and practical support. However, the use of FUR did depend on the PCT agreeing a PBC business plan, alignment of this plan with the strategic objectives of the PCT and, crucially, the availability of PCT resources.

There was some scepticism among interviewees about the role of incentives in encouraging practices to become involved in commissioning. It was argued that it kept GPs away from their practices and there was little profit to be gained. As one interviewee commented:

> 'The most remarkable thing about practice-based commissioning is that anybody does it at all, because there's no profit it ... and certainly no personal gain.' (Director of strategy, site 7)

FUR appeared a substantial incentive in theory, as PCTs could allocate 70% of FUR to practice-based commissioners for developing services. In practice, however, this was dependent on the financial situation of the PCT and was influenced by the extent of overspend in other practices, as well as by the approach adopted by the PCT. All such savings could be withheld. This meant that there was little incentive to develop business plans. One interviewee commented as follows:

> 'We did have a number of GPs quite engaged in practice-based commissioning and that all fell apart in 2007/8 because they were offered the incentive to join up but then they were told during the course of the year there wouldn't be an achievement payment. So there was basically a breakdown in the relationship between the PCT and the practices where they felt, if it's not too strong a word to say, betrayed.' (Director of primary care commissioning, site 1)

The extent to which FUR were targeted towards preventive services was addressed through the study. The effectiveness of FUR was questioned in this context by a number of interviewees, given the annual planning and monitoring cycles which made 'investing to save' difficult, especially as many health and wellbeing initiatives were small-scale pilot projects unlikely to demonstrate effectiveness over the short term. It was difficult to commission services 'off the shelf' or be clear about expected outcomes. In the same way, it was difficult to quantify savings from health promotion or public health interventions and use these resources elsewhere. In contrast, it was clear how money could be released through service reconfiguration. Both the 'pilot nature' of many initiatives and the lack of recurrent funding were considered significant barriers. While there was one example in the case study sites of FUR being used to set up a health café, in a partnership initiative, PBC involvement with the broader health and wellbeing agenda or with identifying the needs of their localities was minimal. One interviewee commented:

> 'But I think by and large practice-based commissioning has not really got to the health and wellbeing agenda. I think it's been very much about service delivery and, you know, community assessment services or joint problems, that kind of thing.' (DPH, site 5)

Neither did the national survey identify many examples of practice-based commissioners commissioning health and wellbeing services from themselves or from other providers, although there were examples of weight management, sexual health and enhanced health checks (from themselves, as providers), and exercise trainers and a traveller outreach project (from other providers). When asked how PCTs were encouraging PBCs to commission health and wellbeing services, the most popular method was through FUR (52%), followed by the use of an innovation fund (34%).

Another barrier was that extra resources could be required to make savings elsewhere in the system.

> 'If I'm going to start saying, well, I will set up a new service internally within the practice to look after all these people in a much more assertive way, and take one of the doctors out of the surgery to do all that ... or I'm going to sit down and pull all these people and review their medication in a much more rigorous way, there is no finance to support that. If I'm going to improve my access sufficiently so that people don't go to A&E, it saves all the money on the budget, but actually I've employed more doctors and nurses to do all

that sort of stuff, and there's no incentive in the system.'
(PEC chair, site 8)

From a system-wide perspective, it was argued that potential savings from service redesign were often less than assumed. Even if progress was made in achieving earlier discharge, for example, new patients would take their place and would be costlier to treat, so it was difficult to release resources from the acute sector. Moreover, while there were incentives for PCTs to manage demand through PBC, as failure to do so would threaten their financial viability, the incentive for NHS Trusts to increase activity resulted in a fundamental imbalance and tension.

Although many interviewees questioned the current emphasis on financial incentives, it was agreed that they acted as a lever for achieving strategic goals. However, they formed only part of the picture and, while the majority of interviewees considered them a spur to action, they needed to be complemented with PCT support for practices. Development support, leadership and management skills were all important, as was benchmarking across practices, demonstration of success and peer approval.

The mixed record of GPs' involvement in commissioning and, in particular, the limited use of FUR to fund preventive services, suggests that involvement required for redesigning services would have been difficult to achieve through the incentives available at the time. However, a lack of time to get involved in commissioning and the difficulties of making savings through managing demand were both raised by interviewees and continue to be debated. There was relatively little involvement by GPs in health needs assessment or in developing a joint preventive health agenda and other studies have demonstrated the relatively limited involvement of PBC in PCT commissioning (Curry et al., 2008). It is not clear how far this is likely to change with the new arrangements, despite the requirement for CCGs to engage with HWBs.

Optional and flexible incentive contracts: local enhanced services

Reviews of the use of incentives in general practice have largely focused on the impact of the QOF (McDonald et al., 2010; Peckham and Wallace, 2010). However, LESs figured prominently in the study and were the most commonly cited vehicle for incentivising preventive activities in GP practices and pharmacies. Introduced in 2004 as part of the new GMS contract, they formed part of a range of enhanced services where incentives could be built in to promote enhanced performance in relation to the QOF or to promote early adoption of new services. They were used to encourage primary care providers to meet local health needs, including the provision of community-based services, and services for underserved groups. They could also be used to incentivise demand management, reducing the use of the acute sector.

Unlike the QOF, LESs are flexible, optional and locally determined service agreements with independent contractors, usually agreed on an annual basis. They were arranged through PCTs at the time of the study and provided an attractive and flexible route through which commissioners could gain a quick response from general practice in addressing local needs or specific targets for delivery. Spending on LESs in England reached a peak of £336 million in 2009/10, but declined to £269.6 million in 2011/12 (Health and Social Care Information Centre, 2013)

From 2013, funding for LESs was included in CCG budgets, with the important exception of preventive LESs, which were rolled into a ring-fenced public health budget, under the control of unitary and upper-tier local authorities. This meant that the variation in the deployment of preventive LESs by PCTs was also carried over. CCGs will be able to fund local schemes to improve the quality of services provided through the GP contract, however.

Views about preventive LESs were sought from national survey respondents and interviewees. These illustrated both the benefits and disadvantages of incentive contracts, the difficulties involved in developing optimal incentive contracts and the importance of balancing solidaristic and extrinsic incentives.

The national survey showed that LESs were the most common vehicle for incentivising activities to reach local targets and were used by 70% of responding PCTs. LESs were also the incentive scheme most often discussed by interviewees. Overall, there were over 150 LESs in the 10 case study sites, with just under half related to preventive services, of which smoking cessation and sexual health services were the most common, followed by cardiovascular risk assessment. Other LESs included falls prevention, care of older people and enhanced services for depression and anxiety, screening for Chlamydia and a 'health inequalities' LES. (A more detailed account of the distribution and range of LESs in case study sites can be found in Marks et al., 2011d.) Payment was either directly related to activity (as for vaccinations, an extension of core services), based on the registered practice population or depended on reaching specific targets. Some LESs included bonus payments or were weighted to encourage targeting of specific populations or areas. Most interviewees agreed that LESs fitted well with what was described as the 'small business' and entrepreneurial model of general practice. They were considered successful in motivating GPs to provide additional services and in pump priming change, although it was also the case that they were the most easily available incentive for commissioners:

> 'I think enhanced services is an interesting area because that's potentially one of the things which enables you to move or see if GP behaviour would move quickly ... amazingly, sometimes when you introduce a LES you can find the capacity appears. So it's about getting the incentive right, but it's being clear [about] what you're getting for that I think.' (Director of strategy, site 7)

LESs had proved useful for meeting national or local targets in relation to smoking and obesity, for example, and for addressing inequalities through cardiovascular screening. They were also seen by PCT interviewees as a way of addressing inadequacies and inflexibilities in the QOF, in particular, proactively identifying populations at risk of premature mortality. Some PCTs chose to weight LESs to encourage targeting of specific populations or areas (in line with the 'incentive intensity' principle). At least two of the ten case study sites had incorporated a public involvement element into their PBC LES and a further PCT wished to develop a LES to support healthy behaviour change through motivational interviewing.

There was evidence of their success. In one example, practices had taken on care for a nursing home, doing 'ward rounds' which had reduced emergency admissions. Smoking cessation targets in one site had been exceeded by creating a LES for general practice that funded a more comprehensive approach to smoking cessation – with dramatic results:

> 'So if the practice now sees a person for the full sort of four to six weeks, they've got the person who's quit smoking and had that confirmed by carbon monoxide testing. Whereas in the past they might have got a fiver for it, they can now get up to hundred and twenty quid for that. All of a sudden, we've gone from missing the target, missing the target, missing target, to so overachieving it, it's amazing. And, you know, these are genuine quitters.' (Director of strategy, site 3)

Despite these advantages, almost half the interviewees levelled criticisms at LESs, raising issues of broader relevance to the deployment of incentives. First of all, they had been developed in an incremental and piecemeal fashion, with some PCTs agreeing large numbers of LESs, where contracts were not always clearly specified or monitored and where there were few sanctions for non-delivery. One interviewee commented:

> 'Because we have ended up in the situation where we have lots of little LESs or contracts that actually we're not performance managing, we don't know what they're delivering in terms of quality, and therefore it's become more of actually you can't tell the difference between what was previously happening and what wasn't. So we've tried to withdraw from those services. Whether I think we need to in the future I think the answer to that is yes, but it goes back to we need to be much better then about how we performance manage and write those contracts.' (DPH, site 8)

In light of this, some PCTs were attempting to consolidate and rationalise the contracts, or channel them through networks rather than individual GPs. More important, however, was the fact that LESs were optional and voluntary, which meant that inequalities in service provision would be increased if targeted practices did not choose to take them up: if large practices did not need additional income they would not be motivated to take advantage of them. Practices could meet their targets for payment but might not have reached the most vulnerable groups and in any event, implementation was patchy:

> 'Enhanced schemes are okay but there's only a finite enhanced services budget; it's not limitless. And if you want to preserve equity at the same time, and if you want to attack health inequalities at the same time, there's no point in setting up an enhanced service that your deployed practices aren't going to take up.' (Practice-based commissioner, site 2)

Some practices were accused of 'cherry picking' LESs, which led one PCT to consider that, instead of individual LESs, they should form part of a wider package across practices. LESs did not reflect a strategic approach: they were often focused on rewarding activity rather than outcomes. Neither was the level of incentive required to achieve improved performance clear. Practices could be receiving rewards for services they were already providing and some practices carried out the same activities for which other practices were being separately incentivised. This meant that LESs were being used to address variability in the level of care provided through general practice.

Interviewees were also ambivalent over the benefits of incentivising through LESs over the longer term, as they were essentially a short-term solution. The incentives designed to stimulate change could become seen as a permanent financial resource:

> 'But, you know, it's about funding change. But then the change becomes the mainstream. If the change doesn't become the mainstream way of working, then you're stuffed, because you're either left with a decision of well we're going to have to incentivise this forever, or we stop incentivising it, and it stops happening.' (DPH, site 4)

Interviewees in a number of sites were not in favour of LESs precisely because they detracted from the values of partnership and encouraged a transactional approach. It was argued that engagement with GPs could prove a more successful route for change and that GPs who were keen innovators were not necessarily interested in financial incentives:

> 'I don't think financial incentives are necessary, I think it's really important to get engagement at a local level first of all ... with our vascular risk policy there is a scheme that will come into effect from next year so that will be focusing on specific areas of our borough. But other GP practices will still be doing those vascular risk assessments without a financial incentive because they do understand how important those things are. So I don't think you necessarily need to throw money to fix the problem.' (PEC chair, site 1)

Moreover, from a system perspective, LESs could often be introduced without regard to implications for increased activity in other parts of the health care system. An example was given of a 'falls LES' that was unsuccessful due to a lack of capacity to respond to referrals from these practices:

> 'If you put an incentive in one part of the system how's the rest of the system aligned to that? Because you can do all the proactive work in the world but if the rest of the system has still only got the capacity to respond to reactive (work) ... it

doesn't take long for the system to get clogged'. (Director of strategic commissioning, site 10) (Marks et al., 2011d: 562)

A number of case study sites were seeking to amend, reduce or package LESs, including clustering related LESs into a Service Level Agreement with general practice networks, encouraging a less piecemeal and more collaborative approach. This could encourage standardisation of care, improve performance management and provide support for weaker practices. Information which allowed practices to benchmark their performance was also a key factor in motivating practices to improve their performance. A more integrated approach would be better incentivised through budgets related to care pathways. Some PCTs considered there would be fewer LESs in future as they were gradually replaced by different contractual arrangements.

LESs raised important issues about what should be considered the core preventive role of general practice, exposed variability in the provision of primary care services – and also in the attempts of commissioners to address these gaps – and highlighted gaps in the QOF. Their use also led interviewees to question the balance across incentives and other sources of motivation

> 'I mean as a doctor myself, I do question do you need to incentivise a professional to do their job they're being paid for, and sometimes I think we overrate the incentive bit and forget about the compelling information, the message, the audit and the feedback to professionals to show the impact of engaging in health and wellbeing.' (Director of strategic planning, site 2) (Marks et al., 2011d: 560)

There were intrinsic satisfactions in doing a job well. A LINk chair noted:

> I have this problem with incentives, in that I believe if somebody's doing a job properly, they should just get on and do it. I hate this thing about I'll pay you if you do this sort of thing. And I think it leads to a concentration on activity rather than outcome.' (Site 3)

Their existence highlighted the fact that evidence-based preventive services were being incentivised through optional arrangements and were not routinely treated as core services. This made them vulnerable to cuts. LESs also illustrated the inadequate consideration of the effect of incentives on the health care system as a whole. Finally, LESs reflected both the advantages and disadvantages of incentive contracts. Problems with LESs reinforce the view that financial incentives need to be considered as part of a wider spectrum of factors motivating change and that incentives cannot be considered in isolation but need to be aligned across a health system. Over the course of the project, there was evidence of a shift from the use of LESs to the use of other contractual flexibilities and more rigorous performance management of primary care.

Despite misgivings over the emphasis on financial incentives, which could undermine intrinsic motivation, interviewees considered them a flexible lever for achieving strategic goals and addressing shortcomings and inflexibilities in the GMS contract. However, a public service ethos and intrinsic motivation were key:

> 'I think that for everybody there is a component of doing the right thing. People want to do a good job and they believe it is worth doing, and I haven't got a more motivational slide [than] the ones showing inequalities and expectation of life by ward.' (Chief executive, site 3)

Non-financial incentives were emphasised in the majority of sites and often associated with 'inspirational leadership'.

> 'Well, the big incentive, and this sounds fluffy and woolly, the incentive here is we understand the needs of the population, and that is a driver, and it's a driver with passion here.' (PCT chair, site 4)

Other sources of motivation, such as peer approval, audit and feedback were also important, and the longer-term cultural change required for general practice to adopt a more proactive approach was unlikely to be achieved through short-term financial incentives.

Moving towards contract specification and alternative providers

Interviewees were often uncertain over the balance to be achieved across incentives and contract specification. Although there was some evidence of declining enthusiasm for using incentives in the first phase of the study, between phases one and two of the fieldwork there was a shift in emphasis from the deployment of incentives to a concentration on contract specification and the performance management of contracts. There was interest in the extent to which contractual arrangements with GPs could be placed on a different footing, including alternative provider medical services (APMS) and personal medical services (PMS) (the latter restricted to medical practitioners) so that performance management arrangements flowed from the nature of the contract. These could be more cost-effective than a large number of LESs. Deployment of contractual levers and contract monitoring for PMS, APMS, and GMS contracts was considered an area for urgent development.

Time-limited APMS contracts offered PCTs greater flexibility, allowing services to be commissioned from a wide variety of sectors, including commercial organisations, voluntary and charitable organisations, social enterprises, mutual providers and public bodies. They could be used for a wide range of services, including services where existing GMS and PMS practices opted out. Their use was becoming increasingly popular as it allowed commissioners to define clearly what was needed from the outset, and they could also include incentives or penalties for not reaching targets agreed in the contract. Recommissioning through APMS (and PMS) could only take place, however, where existing contracts came to an end. The use of APMS (now commissioned nationally through NHS England) increased by 51% in 2010 and a further 5% in 2011 but applies to a small proportion of contracts (Health and Social Care Information Centre, 2013).

The national survey revealed that only 4% of GPs had APMS contracts across the 43 PCTs that responded to this question. In response to a question as to whether PMS and APMS contracts were being specified or reworked explicitly to address health and wellbeing, almost half of the responding PCTs claimed that they were or had these contracts under review. There was far less enthusiasm for APMS among practice-based commissioners in the case studies, as contracts were considered too short term and it could be difficult to remove contracts without leaving populations at risk.

PMS contracts were described as disappointing and not adequately exploited, and there were a number of attempts to ensure that the PMS practices were providing value for money. Contracts needed to be explicit and include health improvement targets:

> 'In terms of our new practices in the PMS-type services, we've been much more explicit about what's within the contract and what we expect them to deliver against and there's clear health improvement targets within those. So I think it's easier to start and put the right things in rather

[than] to look back on the current contracts you have with primary care and change them, because most of them have been in for a long time and GPs are very good at fighting what wasn't in their contract and what is now.' (DPH, site 8)

As mentioned earlier, the emphasis was shifting towards better performance management of PMS contracts and the added value they might bring, and better monitoring of QOF payments, both recognised as relatively neglected areas. The specification of contracts formed part of the governance arrangements which PCTs, as commissioners, needed to put in place. PCTs were increasingly holding practice-based commissioners to account in relation to reducing referrals, non-elective admissions, prescribing budgets and attendances at Accident and Emergency Departments. The movement towards new contractual routes, such as APMS, has been reinforced through the promotion of greater competition in the provision of primary care and preventive services, and is enshrined in the Health and Social Care Act 2012. The highly contested and controversial Section 75 of the Act required commissioners to put out to tender services that could be provided by an organisation other than the NHS, thereby further opening up the NHS to private providers. The extent to which competitive tendering by CCGs is enforced remains to be seen.

Lessons from the research for incentivising service improvement, including preventive services

Many of the findings related to incentives are generic: the importance of considering perverse incentives; assessing potential effects across a whole system; and factors to be considered in developing incentive contracts. In relation to health and health inequalities, the P4P system reflected in the QOF was shown to be lacking and it is not clear to what extent CCGs will seek to overcome its limitations through encouraging proactive case finding and prevention. Since the period of the study, new incentives are being introduced for CCGs to encourage and reward improved quality of care and potential perverse incentives will need to be considered.

Additional resources for health inequalities in baseline budgets were not necessarily targeted towards relevant initiatives unless there was a relevant monitoring system in place (as the lack of impact of the Spearhead monies in the study shows). Specific incentives for providing preventive services through contracts were considered to be effective, even though there were problems in specifying contracts and in monitoring their implementation. However, the existence of so many attempts to incentivise the provision of evidence-based preventive services through GPs illustrated an overall lack of a preventive ethos in primary care. Moreover, preventive initiatives are now commissioned through local authorities, with the original preventive LESs rolled into the ring-fenced public health budget. A range of providers may be commissioned for services such as NHS Health Checks and, while this may include GPs, in a continuation of previous contractual arrangements, it is likely that this balance will change. Issues of contract specification and the inclusion of rewards for delivery or for 'pump priming' change will need to be considered by local authorities as they contract with a range of providers to provide health improvement services. The study showed, for example, how some areas were successfully commissioning services in partnership with the voluntary sector.

Since April 2013, there has been a change in governance arrangements and therefore in system and individual incentives. In a context of austerity, economic incentives are likely to be tied to demand management, which inevitably puts at risk a longer-term preventive agenda. CCGs have direct control of much of the commissioning budget (and are therefore more incentivised to manage demand than was the case with PBC) but also have to meet certain targets in order to receive a quality premium (to be distributed among GPs for improving patient care). This premium involves three local measures and four national measures: reducing avoidable emergency admissions; potential years of life lost from causes considered amenable to health care; rolling out the 'friends and family' test and patient experience of hospital services; and incidence of health care associated infections. However, although the quality premium is broader in scope, some of the difficulties identified in the use of freed up resources [FUR] for practice-based commissioners are likely to persist, as payment of the quality premium requires CCGs to have remained within their resources.

More significant, system incentives remain in conflict and an understanding of the 'science' of incentives remains weak. Kane et al. (2004) point out that incentives do not exist in a vacuum and to be effective they need to be aligned and coordinated across a whole system. The chapter shows that the effectiveness of explicit financial incentives needs further exploration in relation to the context in which they are implemented, their impact on sustained longer-term effects as opposed to short-term changes, the levels at which they should be set and their interrelationship with other motivational factors, including core assumptions over roles and responsibilities. PCTs were able to deploy a wide range of incentives to promote preventive services, however, and it is not clear to what extent these options will be exploited through CCGs or local authorities.

Conclusions

This chapter demonstrates that incentives had limited potential to promote health and wellbeing, that the balance between incentivisation and contract specification (including the nature of core contracts) was changing, and that a transactional approach could undermine engagement and local involvement. Failures in one set of incentives (for example, through the QOF) could be overlaid with additional incentives (QOF plus, or LES). Indicators could be difficult to quantify and monitoring was often inadequate. Incentives could be 'system blind', incentivising increased acute activity or increasing demands on services which were not available. If pitched at the wrong level, incentives could reward what was being done already, or, conversely, demotivate those who were unable to meet the required targets. Failure to meet the requirements of performance management regimes or sanctions arising from poor ratings also acted as incentives to improve performance. However, incentives could lead to perverse consequences and there were possibilities of gaming, paying for services which might have been provided anyway, and an over-reliance on incentives to improve performance and quality of care. Incentives for preventive services also served to underline the failure to systematically implement evidence-based preventive services, replacing them with voluntary schemes which were patchily implemented. Incentives needed to be coupled with longer-term changes in mainstream services.

New approaches to devolved budgets were being considered as a way of increasing a focus on outcomes and a number of interviewees considered that 'collaborative commissioning' was a way forward: for example, one possibility was to involve primary and secondary clinicians within localities based around hospitals, working with social services to manage a budget. Another was to provide a budget through a local network of GPs (through a Service Level Agreement) for a specific pathway of care which would also incorporate preventive services. Networks could also be aligned with local partnership structures to encourage broader partnership working for health and wellbeing, particularly with borough-based services. Another proposition, prefiguring CCGs, was to devolve budgets so that GPs could manage their population's health needs, combined with more control of community services, although it was argued that this model would need to be piloted in order to identify optimal size of budgets and establish collaborative arrangements for sharing risk. Although care pathway development was a common theme, these approaches had different implications for the extent to which practice-based commissioners were likely to become more involved in the health and wellbeing agenda or with local partnerships outside the acute sector. With the advent of CCGs, devolved budgets became a reality, although difficulties in achieving integrated care, joint working on local preventive services or across pathways of care and proactive population-based primary care services remain.

CHAPTER SIX

Prioritising public health investment

> We must re-orientate our health and social care services to focus together on prevention and health promotion. This means a shift in the centre of gravity of spending. (Secretary of State for Health, 2006: 9)

In practice, health systems focus on immediate demands of health care services with, at best, only 3% of the total health expenditure in Organisation for Economic Co-operation and Development (OECD) countries committed to prevention (WHO, 2012a: para. 101). Evidence-based preventive services have not been implemented on the scale required and often fail to reach those most likely to benefit: a wealth of evidence on the health impact of unequal distribution of the social determinants of health has not resulted in effective cross-sector policy action to address inequity, while the tendency to associate public health with population-based preventive services has deflected attention from public health impacts of action in other sectors.

This chapter begins by reviewing arguments for prioritising investment in prevention and then describes initiatives for investing in health developed by the Labour government over the period of the study. It considers views of local stakeholders on enablers for and barriers to investing in prevention and the extent to which interviewees considered that prevention was prioritised in practice. Commitment to principles of 'good governance' is only meaningful if it is reflected in decision-making and priority-setting processes and the chapter assesses approaches to priority setting and decision support in the context of investing in health and addressing health equity. Finally, the impact on priority setting of the relocation of public health to local authorities is discussed.

Prioritising investment in prevention

While the reasons for preventing ill health, reducing health inequalities and increasing healthy life expectancy are primarily ethical and cannot be reduced to an economic balance sheet, costs of avoidable illness to health and other sectors and the scale of action required need to be constantly restated. The World Health Organization (WHO, 2002) quantified more than 25 preventable risks to health and assessed cost-effective measures to reduce them. It showed, for example, that one-third of the disease burden across Europe was caused by tobacco, alcohol, high blood pressure, cholesterol and obesity, and estimated that, in some European countries, life span could increase by about five years if preventive measures were implemented. Across Europe, at least 80% of all heart disease, stroke and Type 2 diabetes and at least one-third of cancer cases are considered preventable (WHO, 2012a). Concern over the scale of preventable morbidity is compounded by its differential distribution across the population. The Commission on Social Determinants of Health (CSDH) documented the stark disparities in life chances within and between countries arising from different social and economic conditions, concluding that 'social injustice is killing people on a grand scale' (WHO, 2008: 26). The social gradient in health underlines the extent of avoidable morbidity and the extent to which it is associated with socioeconomic position, while inequalities between different countries, regions and localities persist. For example, the north of England has experienced a fifth more premature deaths (before the age of 75) than the south and this has persisted over four decades (Hacking et al., 2011). As discussed in the introduction, many reasons have been put forward for the failure to narrow inequalities in health or prioritise the prevention of ill health.

In recent years, recognition of the costs of preventable morbidity to health systems, to sectors outside health and to the wider economy, combined with concerns over the sustainability of health systems, have resulted in greater prominence of economic arguments for investing in health (Merkur et al., 2013). Also emphasised are the substantial economic and social benefits (including improved social cohesion) of a healthy population for society as a whole. *Health 2020* (WHO, 2012a) notes that:

> Investing in health must be seen as an investment in the long-term health and wellbeing of the population as a whole, which is both of intrinsic value and a factor contributing to economic productivity and creating wealth. (para. 625)

Health 2020 noted, for example, the cost-effectiveness of tobacco control programmes, alcohol policies, population-wide action to promote healthy eating and action through the life course to prevent depression. Working in partnership with WHO, a long-term project on the economics of prevention was launched by the OECD in 2007 with the aims of developing a conceptual framework for the economics of non-communicable disease prevention and devising appropriate methods for assessing prevention programmes. In their review of cost-effective public health interventions, Owen et al. (2012) showed that of the public health interventions assessed, the majority were cost-effective (although over 63% of interventions targeted smoking) and by 2014 the Centre for Public Health Excellence at NICE (National Institute for Health and Care Excellence) had produced evidence-based guidance on 52 public health topics which included a costing template to aid with financial planning for implementation.[1] Taking a broader perspective, WHO has launched a project to explore economic rationales for interventions related to the social determinants of health, considering efficiency, equity and value for money. A report on this initiative (WHO, 2013: 10) points out that few value-for-money studies consider equity or 'potential or actual health effects on the benefit side of the equation'.

In England, return on investment debates related to public health were first crystallised in the influential reports of Sir Derek Wanless (2002, 2004). His first report, in 2002, *Securing our future health: Taking a long-term view* (commissioned by HM Treasury) contrasted the costs of preventable ill health with the potential benefits of prevention. Wanless looked at the long term resource requirements for the NHS, and modelled the cost implications of three alternative scenarios (solid progress, slow uptake and fully engaged) for the next 20 years, given various assumptions. This drew attention to the benefits of a healthier population not only through reducing costs of health and social care but also in relation to the wider economy. Public health programmes, implemented effectively, would improve population health and reduce health care costs over the longer term. The report also raised the profile of health-related scenario modelling – modelling health and social care costs and benefits over different time frames.

His second report, *Securing good health for the whole population* (Wanless, 2004) was concerned with the balance between health care and public health measures, and argued for a reorientation of the role of the NHS towards promoting good health, with performance management systems and inspection arrangements to match. He pointed to the 'dearth of evidence of cost-effectiveness' of public health interventions and argued for a combination of predictive modelling (20-year forecasts of the biggest risks to health), analyses of how public health was being organised and decisions taken at both national and local levels, and improvements in the public health evidence base. The report drew attention to the inadequacies of the public health evidence base, failures to assess the impact of government policies on health and the substantial costs of neglecting preventable illness and health inequalities. Wanless also noted the slow acceptance of economic perspectives in public health. While this report was influential, there was disappointment over its lack of longer-term impact, and this was also reflected in the study. One interviewee commented:

'And that's the disappointment really is the government commissioned Wanless, fantastic report, absolutely brilliant. A clean sheet of paper, common sense, financial perspective, economic perspective – what's happened to it? Where is Wanless now?' (Director of public health, site 10)

Since Wanless, there have been further attempts to estimate costs of preventable morbidity for health care and other sectors. In the UK, for example, an estimate of the cost of risk factors for chronic disease (2006/7) showed that ill health related to poor diet cost the NHS £5.8 billion. An update estimated costs of physical inactivity as £0.9 billion, smoking as £3.3 billion and alcohol as £3.3 billion, while overweight and obesity cost £5.1 billion (Scarborough et al., 2011). An estimate of alcohol-related harm (England only) across sectors (Prime Minister's Strategy Unit, 2004) considered costs to the workplace (up to £6.4 billion), health (up to £1.7 billion) and crime and public disorder (up to £7.3 billion). (Costs to families and social networks were unquantified due to data limitations.) The government estimated a total cost in England of £20 billion per annum.

In the period leading up to the study, the Labour government placed greater emphasis on prevention, reflected in advice to commissioners and policy makers to 'to shift the system towards prevention and community based care' (Secretary of State for Health, 2006: 17) and through attempts to strengthen the commissioning process. Commitments to refocus the NHS on prevention were evident in the English Public Health White Paper, *Choosing health* (Secretary of State for Health, 2004) and two years later, in the White Paper, *Our health, our care, our say: A new direction for community services* (Secretary of State for Health, 2006). The *Commissioning framework for health and well-being* (Department of Health, 2007a) paved the way for the world class commissioning (WCC) process and was designed to help commissioners achieve a more strategic orientation towards promoting health, reflected in a stronger focus on commissioning services and interventions across health and local government (para. 1.1). As part of this, there would be flexibility in 'shifting resources to where investment can have the greatest impact on current and future health and wellbeing needs' (para 1.11). Inevitably, spend on prevention needed to be estimated if any shifts in the balance of spending were to be detected. *Are we choosing health?* (Healthcare Commission and the Audit Commission, 2008), also highlighted the importance of identifying resources spent on health improvement and of developing programme budgeting, which was currently inadequate for gauging spend on prevention. This theme was subsequently pursued through Health England, a national reference group for health and wellbeing, set up following *Our health, our care, our say*, where it was noted that:

> At present, the definition and measurement of spend on prevention are not easy to apply. Spend on prevention and spend on public health should be separated more clearly. International and UK definitions of preventative and public health spend are not aligned, and issues like service quality are not adequately captured. (para. 6.34)

These remarks were prescient, given the difficulties in calculating the public health budget to be transferred from the NHS to local authorities from April 2013.

From 2007 until it was wound up in 2009, Health England produced reports estimating preventive health spend (PHS) to support an evidence-based shift to preventive services. (Health England, 2007, 2009). It demonstrated wide variation in spend across primary care trusts (PCTs) and argued that spend in a country or locality should be related to levels of morbidity or mortality and new national service frameworks (NSFs) should include plans for monitoring spend and the effectiveness of preventive actions. However, there were difficulties over the breadth of the public health agenda and, therefore, over what should be included and measured as part of PHS. The attempts to identify the NHS spend on prevention prior to transferring it to local authorities exposed extensive variation in how much PCTs had spent per head on prevention and, while attempts were made to provide a fairer distribution, the allocation decisions made were controversial (House of Commons Communities and Local Government Committee, 2013).

While ethical, practical and methodological issues have been well rehearsed in relation to priority setting in health care, there has been far less emphasis on priority setting in social care or in public health, despite the scale and cost of preventable ill health. At a local level, in England, there were attempts to demonstrate the benefits to commissioners of investing in preventive initiatives. For example, based on historic provision (and therefore open to improvement), an example for PCTs cited in Bernstein et al. (2010) showed a local return on investment which was over double the cost of interventions related to smoking, alcohol and obesity (taken as a whole). There were also attempts to encourage commissioners to adopt economic thinking in priority setting, including a shift in the balance across prevention and treatment, often in the context of rebalancing services across a pathway of care. More recently, studies have focused on assessing the relevance to public health investment of priority-setting methods typically used for rationing health care (Matrix Insight, 2011; Morgan et al., 2011; Marks et al., 2013a). The business case for local authority engagement in health improvement has been assessed (Matrix Insight, 2009a), along with support for implementation (Matrix Insight, 2011). Criteria for assessing priorities need to be transparent if commissioners are to be held accountable and transparency is even more important where difficult decisions need to be made over disinvestment: transparent priority-setting methods therefore form part of good governance for commissioners. With the transfer of public health into local authorities, social return on investment, which incorporates social, environmental and economic costs and benefits into decision making, is likely to become more prominent and is consistent with adopting a broader public health approach and a longer-term perspective.

The WCC assurance system (Department of Health, 2008a), described in more detail in Chapter Three, had a tripartite assurance system covering health outcomes, commissioning competencies and governance requirements. As part of this, competencies in priority setting, and in ensuring efficiency and effectiveness of total expenditure were emphasised. Competency six was described as follows:

> By having a clear understanding of the needs of different sections of the local population, PCTs with their partners will set strategic priorities and make investment decisions, focused on the achievement of key clinical and other outcomes. This will include investment plans that address areas of greatest health inequality. (Department of Health, 2008a: 80)

Indicators included predictive modelling and scenario planning, prioritisation of investment to improve population health and an understanding of return on investment and disinvestment. Part of the requirement for meeting level four (the highest level) in the WCC assessment scale related to the competencies was that 'the PCT invests for longer-term health gain and can quantify impact'.

Related to competency six was competency 11, to 'make sound financial investments to ensure sustainable development and value for money'. It focused on efficiency and effectiveness of total expenditure and on developing a proactive approach to budgeting, including programme budgeting, in order to understand 'investment against outcomes'. The focus on health gain across all spend therefore provided an important change in emphasis, aligned with a concentration on 'allocative efficiency', that is, using resources as a whole to their most beneficial effect.

Influences on prioritising prevention: views from the study

At the time of the study, priority setting had gained a higher profile, partly as a result of its being included in WCC competencies, partly in recognition of the relatively poor performance of commissioning organisations in this respect and, more specifically, in the context of directives to increase productivity and get the best value out of the resources available, while at the same time improving quality.

In relation to public health investment, interviewees and survey respondents identified a wide range of influences. These included national policy guidance, the WCC assurance framework (including the two mandatory health outcomes related to improving health and addressing health inequalities), local health needs identified through the joint strategic needs assessment (JSNA), independent annual DPH (director of public health) reports, national and local targets and the results of public consultation. Alignment of financial planning and strategic aims, as required through the WCC process, was seen as an important lever. Other enablers for a public health agenda included the adoption of a public health approach to the commissioning process as a whole and committed leadership and high level support. The PCT board was considered to play a key role in influencing values which informed the emphasis on health and wellbeing in the PCT and criteria used in prioritisation processes. As discussed in Chapter Three, the majority of interviewees cited the chief executive, the DPH or the board in this respect, stating, for example, that board commitment and 'leadership from the top' had been a significant lever for investing in health and wellbeing:

> 'I've been here now nearly five years, and it's the only organisation I've ever come to where absolutely everybody,

including the board, believe that the only way that we're going to reduce health inequality and increase health and wellbeing is to do things differently and to put more emphasis on upstream work, and they just get it.' (Deputy chief executive, site 8)

Leadership of DsPH was important in 'engaging the whole organisation'. The national survey reflected this emphasis, with 90% of respondents locating priority setting at board level, and 70% citing the role of the DPH.

The influence on priorities exerted by GPs (through PBC [practice-based commissioning]) and by the public (see Chapter Seven for further discussion) was variable. Some interviewees from PBC consortia considered the process centrally controlled: while priorities might have been agreed by PBC clusters, it was less clear how these decisions then influenced the PCT prioritisation process or the annual operating plan. In other sites, practice-based commissioners were highly involved:

'They were involved in determining what the criteria were, what the weighting should be. We basically involve them in everything. We have a very proactive PBC group ... we don't have to drag them to the table, put it that way.' (Finance director, site 9)

PBC leads were often involved in prioritising across a particular programme or pathway of care, examining the cost-effectiveness of each initiative, sometimes segmented by different groups and including some consultation with the community. The preventive element of pathway redesign was less developed and redesign was also made more difficult where aspects of the pathway were outside the remit of the commissioner or where information was required from other organisations.

However, interviewees identified many barriers to public health investment, including the lack of an evidence base for demonstrating return on investment (raised in each case study site). They commented on limited evidence for the effectiveness of public health programmes when there was increased pressure to demonstrate the business case, not just for new health improvement initiatives but also for established services. Acute sector priorities dominated the decision-making process and an emphasis on short-term targets worked against a longer-term public health agenda. Finally, health improvement initiatives were typically funded from growth money and the financial crisis cast doubt on the extent to which such initiatives could be continued. Table 6.1 shows the range of views reflected in case study sites (numbers indicate the number of sites [total 10] where these views were expressed).

National survey respondents also identified barriers to commissioning for health and wellbeing (Figure 6.1). Pressure from acute budgets was viewed as the greatest barrier (by 84 PCTs). Financial pressures were next (59 PCTs), followed by the emphasis on short-term gains (50 PCTs) which worked against a public health perspective.

Despite these barriers, the early period of the study saw a growth in investment for health and wellbeing. The national survey showed that a majority of responding PCTs had increased their investment in 2008/9 compared with 2007/8, largely instigated by strategic decisions taken at board level, SHA level or in partnership with local authorities. Investment was directed to 'upstream' interventions, preventive care or reducing demand in secondary care. The main strategies through which the majority of PCTs in the study intended to shift investment towards health and wellbeing was through growth money and, to a lesser extent, through efficiency savings (see Figure 6.2). Interviewees also emphasised the importance of growth money for the ability to invest in health promotion and in services to reduce health inequalities.

By the time of second-phase interviews (2009/10) questions of efficiency, prioritisation, achieving value for money in more clearly specified contracts, and the development of tools for prioritising investment and disinvestment had gained in importance, although it was recognised by interviewees that modelling skills needed to be developed.

One interviewee noted improvements in how such decisions were being reached:

> 'I remember... there was a pile of like commissioning proposals, and we had one hour, and then there were some providers around the table, and some commissioners and providers were very vociferous, and it was just kind of like all right that one, no why that one? ... if the public had seen that then that would just be appalling, and then last year we had a process which was quite good.' (Assistant DPH, site 5)

In a context of austerity, decisions would need to be made over disinvestment across total spend (sometimes referred to as 'recommissioning in a different way' or 'optimising resources'). Without disinvestment in acute care and reductions in prescribing costs, it would be difficult to fulfil strategic priorities, including those related

Table 6.1: Prioritising investment in public health in 10 NHS commissioning organisations in England

Impact of WCC on priority setting	Governance and priority setting	Prioritising growth funds/efficiency savings	Approaches to rebalancing investment	Priority-setting problems	Enabling factors for prioritising prevention	Barriers	Ways forward
Priorities are based on health needs assessments (10)	Corporate governance / performance management should be aligned to strategic priorities (8)	Plans are scored against national and local targets (10)	Identify outliers (in cost and outcomes) through benchmarking using national data (10)	Rationale and methods for weighting criteria in prioritisation matrices(6)	Leadership/commitment of board and of Executive directors to the health of the population and to addressing health inequalities (10)	Evidence base for ROI of preventive interventions needs development (10)	Develop business cases for public health and demonstrate ROI for public health interventions over different time periods (10)
The commissioning cycle is linked to a national assurance process (10)	Partnerships are required to fulfil the stewardship role (8)	Business plans are aligned with health needs assessments and with strategic priorities (10)	Redesign services to release efficiencies within (9) and across (4) pathways of care	Data for programme budgeting is out of date/poor quality/requires disaggregation (4)	Commissioning cycle is public health-led (8)	Short termism in national policy (10)	Develop skills in public health priority setting (6) (epidemiology, health economics, demography and risk analysis (1) and predictive modelling/ scenario planning (4))
Organisational structures have been changed to reflect the commissioning process (8)	Public is involved in local health needs assessment (7) and in priority- setting (5)	Business plans ranked by (weighted) assessment criteria (e.g. cost-effectiveness, health inequalities) (10)	Disinvestment strategies are in place (3) or planned (7)	Disinvestment skills are lacking (5) and disinvestment strategies can lead to public opposition (2) and threaten viability of hospitals(2)	WCC encouraged the development of explicit prioritisation processes (7), a focus on health outcomes (5) and longer-term perspective (4)	Performance management and incentives prioritise short-term priorities/ process targets in acute sector (9)	Consider value for money across total NHS budget (5) and across health and local authorities (1)

Impact of WCC on priority setting	Governance and priority setting	Prioritising growth funds/efficiency savings	Approaches to rebalancing investment	Priority-setting problems	Enabling factors for prioritising prevention	Barriers	Ways forward
Strategic and financial plans are aligned (6)	Accountability for achieving ROI for population health (6) / awareness of opportunity cost (2)	Preventive services are funded from growth funds once financial balance is achieved (9)	Scenario modelling (3)	Lack of rigour in prioritisation processes (3)	Policy emphasis on a preventive agenda (4)	The wider determinants of health are outwith NHS control (8) and evidence base is complex (1)	Provide ROI data to local GP practices so they can target preventive activities (2)
	Applying the principle of social equity (1)	Prioritisation pro formas, matrices and ethical frameworks have been developed (8)	PBMA /decision conferencing used to assess opportunity costs (2)	Lack of public involvement in decision making over priorities (2)	Setting ring-fenced preventive budgets (3)	Public is more concerned with treatment services (8)	Better understanding of costs of prevention and treatment across pathways of care (2)
			Consider balance of investment across prevention and treatment within and across all programmes of care, and across the total budget (2)	Economic skills are lacking (6). PBMA is time consuming/difficult (1)	Short-term return on investment for preventive initiatives has been demonstrated (3)	Preventive spend is difficult to define or identify as a baseline (8). This makes ROI difficult to assess (1)	Develop Health Impact Assessment in local authorities (1)
			Rebalancing investment through annual percentage increase in prevention budgets (1)			Preventive services are 'easy targets' for cuts (5)	Recognise that priority setting is not just a technical but a political exercise (1)
						NICE Guidelines distort balance of spend to acute sector (1)	

Source: Phase one interviews with PCT decision makers from 10 case study sites (numbers in brackets refer to PCTs). (Reprinted from Marks et al, 2013a, Copyright 2013, with permission from Elsevier)..

Figure 6.1: Barriers to commissioning for health and wellbeing

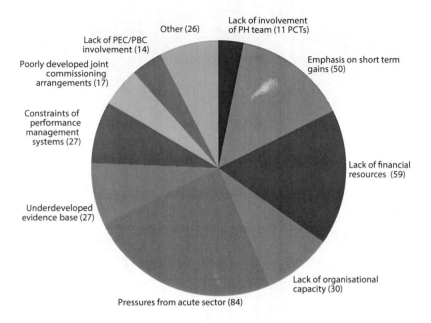

Source: Marks et al. (2011a: 111).

Figure 6.2: Strategies for shifting investment

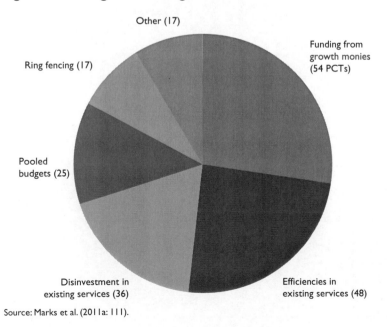

Source: Marks et al. (2011a: 111).

to health promotion, even if return on investment in preventive care could be demonstrated:

> 'It's very easy to do it when you've got lots of new money, but the reality is there isn't lots of new money, so what you have to do is you have to look at where are you going to disinvest to invest. And although the health service talks about disinvestment, to date there is a limited track record of disinvestment I would say. What there has been is a holding, a control of cost to a level, but it's never been about stopping things and reducing things, and one of the things we have to get into now is disinvesting.' (Director of operations, site 8)

There was widespread scepticism over the ability of commissioners to disinvest in existing services, an area where there was limited experience. There would be public and possibly political opposition, resistance from the acute sector and a risk of destabilising the local health economy. In contrast, reducing spending on health and wellbeing was a 'soft option' given that it was 'invisible', benefits were long term and, unlike changes to health care provision, it did not lead to a public outcry:

> 'You know, there are not ten thousand disappointed people who are fed up because they're not getting something to stop them getting bronchitis or lung cancer in five or ten years' time.' (DPH, site 5 in Marks et al., 2013a: 413)

A number of interviewees noted that preventive services, including vascular checks and referral to Weight Watchers, had already been cut back and there was pressure to assess all interventions, including existing services, in relation to their outcomes for the population and their cost-effectiveness.

> 'They will drop off the bottom of the list, and all we can do is continue to look for cost-effective ways of doing it but, you know, for us especially in the next year or two we've really got to target those areas where we can get most money back out of the system... unless we get those right now and get the big chunks of money out of the system, we won't be able to afford to do the health and wellbeing agenda.' (Director of quality, site 9)

Other interviewees were of the opinion that the economic downturn would also prevent the piloting of innovative approaches which could be mainstreamed if effective. While the dominant view was that the health and wellbeing agenda was under threat, it was also argued that commissioners should not be storing up problems for the future by neglecting health improvement. A few interviewees saw some potentially positive aspects of the current climate: for example, economic stringency could act as a spur for radical restructuring as well as for prevention and 'investing to save'. Financial pressures might even encourage 'whole system' thinking:

> 'But I think the financial pressure might actually help us to think as a whole system, and that's certainly the position we're trying to get to here locally is how do we start changing the pathway and upstreaming services, so we can have the community focus on early intervention and our key partners are very much part of that. It's not easy obviously because everybody organisationally needs to keep their services well resourced but everyone recognises that's the change that we have to deliver.' (Director of strategic commissioning, site 10)

In the same way, it was argued that the Department of Health QIPP (Quality Innovation, Productivity and Prevention) programme, introduced in 2010 and designed to save £20 billion by 2014–15, could encourage a creative approach to partnership and to developing care pathways across health and social services, with the aims of avoiding duplication, improving efficiency and avoiding transfer problems. The national survey also identified some positive views: for a small number of respondents, tightened budgets would mean an opportunity to tackle acute spend and plan disinvestment. Furthermore, a few respondents argued that a shift 'upstream' was gaining greater attention as a means of maximising return on investment. Interviewees in a majority of the case study sites argued for further development of decision support tools, including public health modelling with economic projections, in order to demonstrate return on investment.

The following section summarises the range of approaches to priority setting for public health, an area which commissioners considered poorly developed, before considering the decision-making approaches used in practice by commissioners in the study.

Approaches to priority setting for public health

A review of decision support tools was carried out as part of the study, in order to provide a context for the views of local commissioners and to assess the relevance of these tools for public health investment. In England, there is no formal process for prioritising investment. While NICE provides guidance based on evidence of cost-effectiveness of interventions, which includes public health interventions, there is no overt process for ranking interventions, identifying cost-impact, or assessing the implications for disinvestment that may arise as a result of implementing new guidance. In a context of austerity these priority-setting choices become starker, transparency becomes even more important and investment strategies will need to be accompanied by disinvestment strategies. In general, commissioners aim to ensure that each programme or intervention represents an efficient use of resources and that, taken together, these maximise total health benefits, subject to budgetary and resource constraints. They will need to take account of different (and sometimes conflicting) goals such as promoting equity, achieving efficiency of spend, reflecting community views, and reaching a balance between responding to immediate demands and promoting longer-term health gains. Costs and benefits across different sectors may be relevant and, in order to demonstrate transparency in decision making, they need to describe and quantify the uncertainty associated with decisions and the assumptions underlying them.

Decisions over public health investment are influenced by whether the aim is to prioritise within an overall budget for preventive services, shift the balance of spending towards prevention across a pathway of care (for the NHS) or within and across different sectors (in a local authority context), or to increase the proportion of resources for preventive services and approaches across the system as a whole. These decisions are influenced by national and local priorities, the balance adopted across clinical interventions and action related to wider determinants of health, and the priorities of local partnerships.

This section considers priority setting for public health in two stages. The first stage is public health intelligence that helps inform the choice of priority areas and also informs criteria for choosing between different options and interventions. For example, criteria related to prioritising across public health interventions and for public health investment more broadly are likely to include some combination of the following:

- cost–impact (overall cost of implementing an intervention);
- cost–effectiveness of the intervention (as measured by cost per quality of life year [QALY], see below);
- effects on health equity, premature mortality rates, and the overall level of preventable morbidity;
- relevance to social determinants of health and health equity;
- a consideration of impact over different time periods (see modelling section, below);
- longer-term perspectives, required for public health approaches;
- acceptability;
- return on investment (in financial terms) and social return on investment which also includes social and environmental costs and benefits, as part of estimating social value;
- potential costs and benefits in other sectors (see, for example, Morgan et al., 2011).

The range of criteria involved in public health investment has implications not just for the type of economic evaluation and prioritisation methods to be adopted but also for the partnerships involved in decision making. A review of criteria used in health care decision making showed that equity and fairness were the most frequently reported criteria (although difficult to operationalise), followed by efficacy and effectiveness (Guindo et al., 2012). Feeding into these public health investment debates is evidence on addressing inequalities in health and the evidence-based policy priorities developed through the strategic review of health inequalities in England (Marmot Review, 2010) (see Chapter Three).

A second stage is reaching decisions which are transparent and where accountability can be demonstrated. There is a range of generic priority-setting tools which encourage transparency in making choices in the context of selected criteria and the majority can (but do not always) involve the public through methods such as decision conferencing (Airoldi et al., 2011). While these tools have largely been used for prioritising in health care settings, the relevance of specific tools (or combinations of tools) for decision support for public health investment has to be separately and critically assessed. These two stages are discussed in turn.

Public health intelligence: informing the choice of priority areas and criteria for assessment

As discussed earlier, local priorities for improving population health and addressing health inequalities will reflect health needs reflected in JSNAs, national priorities and guidance, and data on relative performance on key public health outcomes, such as levels of premature mortality. JSNAs, and the joint health and wellbeing strategies which build on them, draw on a range of demographic, epidemiological, lifestyle and socioeconomic data (as described in Chapter Three), as well as local views. One interviewee described a public health-led approach to developing priorities:

> 'And the criteria would be public health criteria in the main, i.e. the prevalence of the disease, the importance of the disease, in terms of burden ... the distribution of health needs by economic group, by ethnic group, by area, the cost-effectiveness of the existing treatments, the analysis of the existing service, and the gap between the existing service and the service you want, and so on and so forth.' (DPH, site 1 in Marks et al., 2013a:)

Epidemiological, economic and modelling skills are all required for identifying local public health priorities and for developing local JSNAs and joint health and wellbeing strategies. These are in addition to the information requirements and data sets for JSNAs discussed in Chapter Three. Box 6.1 illustrates public health intelligence relevant for prioritising public health investment. This draws on study findings, which assessed public health intelligence and priority-setting tools against 23 criteria relevant to achieving competencies 6 and 11 of the WCC assurance framework. These criteria included equity, ease of use and public involvement (Marks et al., 2011a): commissioners need to take account of views of the public and stakeholder groups on public health and health care priorities, access to services and future strategies, although the extent to which this occurred in the study was variable (see Chapter Seven). Despite requirements for commissioners to be both accountable and transparent, the study showed that skills in using prioritisation methods, including modelling, were in short supply within PCTs at the time of the study.

Box 6.1: Using public health intelligence

Burden of illness studies estimate leading causes of preventable illness, premature mortality and disability for defined populations and can be used to benchmark performance, track changes over time and model the likely prevalence of preventable illness or disability (overall or for specific diseases) (Capewell et al., 2008). The burden of preventable illness can be estimated across a region and compared with preventative health spend, to help indicate the degree of alignment, or misalignment across public health priorities and spending decisions. The ongoing WHO Global Burden of Disease project,[2] established in 1990, assesses burden of disease based on DALYs (disability-adjusted life years), which measure years of life lost from premature death and years of life lived in less than full health.

Assessment of performance against public health indicators may be included under the four domains of the public health outcomes framework, namely the wider determinants of health; health improvement; health protection; and healthcare and premature mortality (Department of Health, 2012a). This framework provides scope for benchmarking and learning from good practice.

Evidence based on the social determinants of health and health equity: Commissioners need to take account of the social determinants of health and the inequalities in health associated with their distribution (Whitehead and Popay, 2010) and how these are reflected in local socioeconomic and geographical health inequalities. They can also carry out health equity audit of existing policies (Joffe and Mindell, 2005); health impact assessment of new policies (Kemm and Parry, 2004); and health equity impact assessment (Povall et al., 2013).

Costs of preventable illnesses or health damaging behaviours across health care, other sectors and the wider economy: Estimates of the economic burden of preventable morbidity across sectors including, but not limited to, the costs to the NHS, provide a basis for partnerships to address risk factors, including smoking, obesity and drug and alcohol misuse as well for estimating the return on investment from preventive activities.

Identifying, measuring and tracking preventative spend (as a measure of overall spend and within programmes of care: Preventative health spend has proved difficult to identify and define (Secretary of State for Health, 2006: para. 6.34) but without it, the priority afforded to prevention (or signs of a shift towards it) may be difficult to track or monitor.

Benchmarking: This allows for the comparison of outcomes for similar organisations. Quadrant Analysis can be used to compare health outcome and expenditure data on a single cost-effectiveness type plane (higher/lower spend, higher/lower outcome). For example, SPOT (spend and outcome tool) was developed to help PCTs (and then CCGs) identify outlier programmes, that is, programmes with health outcomes and/or expenditure substantially different from the average (Yorkshire and Humber Health Intelligence, n.d.). Public Health England provides standardised, benchmarked information relevant for JSNAs and joint health and wellbeing strategies.

Public health investment also requires a longer-term and anticipatory approach. Modelling the impact of public health activities can therefore play a key role in public health investment. There are many different types, including the following, although their use by local commissioners may depend on access to interactive tools which simply require local data input:

- Modelling the impact on outcomes over time of specific public health interventions. As one example of this, the Health Inequalities Intervention Toolkit (Association of Public Health Observatories and Department of Health, n.d.) provides an interactive resource for estimating the impact of high-impact interventions on narrowing the gap in life expectancy (that is, smoking cessation, interventions to reduce infant mortality, treatment for hypertension, treatment with statins and lowering high blood sugar). It allows investigation of effects across the local authority or in the most deprived quintile. This tool was initially developed to help PCTs meet the national health inequalities target.
- Modelling the impact on costs and benefits over different time horizons of alternative strategies for prevention and treatment (Davies et al., 2004). This can also be applied across a pathway of care for a specific condition.
- Scenario planning, where health outcomes over specified time periods are modelled in relation to levels of investment. For example, the use of 'scenario generator', a modelling tool, allows simulation of whole health and social care systems and is configured with prevalence data and with a number of generic pathways of care.[3]
- Predictive models showing the extent and direction of travel of major preventable health problems and associated costs. These can be used for planning and commissioning purposes. Predictive risk models can be used to identify those at risk of unplanned hospital admission and target investment for preventive measures (Lewis et al., 2011).

- Disease prevalence modelling can be used to estimate diseases or risk factors where direct evidence is not available. It can also be used to support proactive case finding where levels of recorded illness are lower than expected.[4]

Choosing between options

Once options for meeting priorities have been identified, criteria for choosing between them have to be agreed and different options assessed, with selected (usually multiple) criteria weighted and scored so that the various options can be ranked. This typically involves data input as well as views of stakeholders. Adopting such a process encourages transparency and clarity over assumptions underlying decisions and makes opportunity costs explicit.

Decision support methods vary in terms of complexity, resources, skills and information required, and there are a number of reviews of priority-setting tools which set out their relative benefits and disadvantages (Williams et al., 2012; Marks et al., 2013b). Most tools can be applied at different levels but all are subject to uncertainty and are aids to decision making only.

Tools include the various methods for economic evaluation, including cost-effectiveness, cost-benefit, cost-consequence and cost-utility analysis, and forms of multi-criteria decision analysis (MCDA) which help decision makers consider multiple criteria, including economic evaluations, in a rational and consistent way. Surveys or paired comparison analysis may be used to identify trade-offs across decision criteria, which are likely to occur where different principles or criteria (such as equity and efficiency) are in conflict. MCDA may be used to develop scorecards, in option appraisal and in programme budgeting and marginal analysis (PBMA). The latter was particularly promoted through WCC and is a pragmatic, priority-setting aid to identify how resources are being spent before exploring potential changes in service provision at the margin, in order to maximise benefit and minimise cost (Ruta et al., 2005). The first stage, programme budgeting, involved identifying (i) the total resources/funds available and (ii) the services these funds were being spent on in each of 23 broad areas based on the WHO International Classification of Diseases (version 10). The second stage, marginal analysis, involved making choices across interventions/programmes at the margins. In general, PBMA is used to examine the benefit gained from an additional unit of resources or the benefit lost from having one unit less.

There are also other approaches. For example, population cost-impact approaches are used to present the benefits and costs for a particular population of moving from current to best practice. They involve three key steps: (i) determining the number of events potentially preventable over a set time; (ii) for the relevant intervention(s), calculating costs to derive cost per event prevented; and (iii) obtaining decision makers' preferences for one population impact measure over another based on a ranking procedure or a valuation exercise. The decision maker is asked to choose between alternative interventions for the highest ranked items.

One of the key criteria informing the choice of priorities (as well as for choosing between them) is evidence of cost-effectiveness. There are numerous resources on cost-effective public health interventions available to commissioners, including:

- NICE public health guidance and commissioning guides provide guidance, costing templates, business cases and recommendations for populations and individuals on activities, policies and strategies that can help prevent disease or improve health. These include methods for assessing cost-effectiveness, cost-impact and return on investment. NICE also produces briefings for local government and members of health and wellbeing boards (HWBs).
- The Health England Leading Prioritisation Tool (Matrix Insight, 2009b) is an online tool that can be used interactively to obtain information on the cost-effectiveness and impact on health inequalities for 17 interventions comprising programmes related to alcohol use, mental health, obesity, smoking cessation and sexually transmitted infections.
- The Public Health Interventions Cost-effectiveness Database (PHICED) is an online, electronic database of bibliographic records related to public health.[5]

A prioritisation exercise, carried out in the USA, involved a systematic review of the effectiveness, cost-effectiveness (using QALYs) and also the preventable burden of disease for 25 clinical preventive services (identified by the US Preventive Services Task Force and the Advisory Committee on Immunisation Practices) when targeted to 90% of the relevant population (Maciosek et al., 2006). However, it did not explicitly include equity considerations and stakeholders, such as the public or service users, were not involved in this exercise (Fox-Rushby et al., 2008).

There are long standing debates over the relevance of cost-effectiveness or cost-utility measures for prioritising public health investment as a whole (as opposed to choosing cost-effective interventions) and over the relative benefits of QALYs (which combine life expectancy and quality of life) and DALYs (disability-adjusted life years, which include years of life lost and years lived with a disability) which have been considered to be more appropriate for informing investment decisions (Health England, 2007). It has been argued that, while QALYs are appropriate measures for assessing public health interventions, overall benefits across a total budget for preventive programmes might be better measured through assessing years of life lost or through DALYs (as used in the WHO Global Burden of Disease project). However, the limitations of cost-utility analysis for public health investment extend further than this. In a briefing document on public health economic evaluation, Kelly et al. (2005: 1) acknowledged that 'the economic appraisal of public health interventions is both underdeveloped and intrinsically difficult'. They point out that the evidence base is skewed towards single initiatives and downstream interventions and that it is difficult to distinguish cause and effect where interventions are multifaceted or community based, with effects only evident over the longer term. While 'cost per QALY' estimates, already used within the more clinical aspects of public health, show that public health interventions compare favourably with treatment interventions, they are not an adequate outcome measure for the complexity of public health interventions. They are difficult to apply to complex upstream interventions, do not usually include non-health sector costs and do not consider equity impacts, that is, issues of distribution of health benefits across a population. Upstream interventions which improve the circumstances in which people live may have a range of beneficial outcomes but only have a limited impact for specific public health targets such as smoking cessation rates. They may, therefore, be hard to evaluate and justify as value for money within this context. Moreover, as mentioned earlier, methods of evaluation adopted by NICE do not take account of the burden of disease. A study of decision making for public health by local decision makers, including local authorities (Morgan et al., 2011) showed that the metric (cost per QALY) was little used. It was argued that cost-benefit analysis (which takes account of the population affected) would be more relevant for decision makers. Clearly, interventions with similar cost-effectiveness (as reflected in the cost of health gain) can have very different impacts on overall costs.

An extensive review of economic evaluations of public health interventions (Drummond et al., 2007, 2008) showed that studies seldom considered non-health sector costs and consequences. There was a tendency towards shorter-term or process outcomes rather than longer-term generic health outcomes. A systematic review to determine the extent to which different methods of economic evaluation have been applied to public health interventions (McDaid and Needle, 2008) showed that only 5% were cost-benefit analyses (the most established approach for evaluating complex multi-agency interventions) and few studies looked at the economic case for tackling the wider determinants of health. Overall, equity considerations across populations were seldom considered and not addressed formally. The review of methodology identified the need for debate over current forms of economic evaluation and recommended that the intersectoral impact of interventions should be quantified using cost-consequence analysis. Claxton and colleagues (2007) discuss some of the issues that arise in trying to generalise health economic methods into public health, and in evaluating costs and effects across sectors, with differing objectives and constraints, and favour a 'compensation test' for public health interventions with multiple outcomes and intersectoral effects.

Commissioners therefore need to consider assumptions which may be built in to specific approaches to decision support, the relative costs and benefits of different tools and the combination of decision support methods most appropriate for specific issues, for involving the public, or for maximising health gain over time. Important considerations include the extent to which decision support approaches incorporate modelling techniques for assessing costs and benefits over the longer term, assess the balance of investment across total spend, assess equity issues, and incorporate intersectoral impact. For example, cost-benefit analysis rarely considers equity issues and PBMA has largely been used in prioritising health care resources. Moreover, most decision support methods have been used for investment of new resources rather than for disinvestment, and many do not model costs and benefits over time. A focus on the cost-effectiveness of specific interventions may work against broader public health investment strategies. Although decisions about the balance of investment across total spend raises additional issues to prioritising across interventions, the quality of predictive modelling and scenario generation partly rests on evidence of cost-effectiveness of public health interventions.

Views expressed by interviewees over prioritisation methods

Discussion of prioritisation methods was mainly limited to PCT interviewees, who described a range of methods for allocating growth funds or for shifting the balance of investment across programmes. New proposals were typically prioritised through locally developed approaches, although these were often described as 'just a spreadsheet' and in the process of development. The process was similar across all case study sites: proposals were developed, scored against national targets, local targets and priorities in the strategic plan, following which a business case was developed and the proposal further scrutinised and weighed up against other investments. Public health investment would be subject to the same rigour as any other area in relation to proving the business case. Most PCTs used a prioritisation matrix, gateway process or ethical framework to aid decision making. These included varying numbers of criteria which might or might not include longer-term benefits. Processes were being refined and weighted criteria applied to initiatives, often as a result of stakeholder involvement. Many interviewees noted that local tools had been developed for this purpose, but it was recognised that further work was needed. One PCT commissioner noted:

> 'Ultimately we come down to what's the total cost being put forward in this particular bid, what number of people will it benefit and therefore what's the cost per beneficiary. What we haven't done is weight the level of benefit. Is it life saving? Is it a quality of life investment? And that, if you like, we haven't done that sort of weighting of the benefit really; it's quite crude, in other words.' (Director of strategy, site 3 in Marks et al., 2013a: 415)

Programme budgeting was widely used: other approaches included prioritising interventions across the life course; prioritising in relation to different scenarios (not limited to financial scenarios but also including changes in demography and patterns of health and illness); and prioritising across scenarios jointly developed with local authorities.

Case study findings were borne out by the national survey which showed use of prioritisation matrices (92% of PCTs), while over 80% used health inequality intervention tools, NICE costing tools and programme budgeting. Around 25% of PCTs responding to the survey appeared to have developed their own tools, with most mentioning their own modified prioritisation tools, while other PCTs mentioned the importance of the JSNA, value for money, WCC processes and tools designed to 'calculate the impact of preventive interventions'. As mentioned earlier, a common approach was to use national programme budgeting data as a benchmarking tool in order to identify outlier areas, compared with the PCT cluster, as priorities for investigation and possible sources of savings. A finance director described the process as follows:

> 'If you happen to be an outlier in terms of cost, but you're getting really good outcomes too, then actually that's not such a bad thing. But if you're an outlier in cost and your outcomes are worse than maybe your cluster group, who are getting better outcomes for less money, then what is it that they're doing that we're not?' (Site 9 in Marks et al., 2013a: 415)

This process was useful where cost-effectiveness data were not available: investigating outliers could sharpen up the prioritisation process and could demonstrate areas where there could be a payback from preventive services and from primary care.

Programme budgeting was also described as being helpful for investing upstream for each programme. Stakeholders, including practice-based commissioners, described initiatives to prioritise across programmes and patient pathways, examining the cost-effectiveness of each initiative in relation to the effect on morbidity and mortality, possibly segmented by different groups and including some consultation with the community. One site had developed a 'clinical economic pathway process' which segmented care pathways, identified current spend, analysed evidence of effectiveness and determined the impact of further investment on the whole pathway. The point was also made that questions should be raised about the balance of resources across different programmes of care and across total spend, as well as within specific programme budget areas, which already reflected implicit priorities over spending in relation to different areas of care.

As mentioned above, while programme budgeting was considered a valuable technique in principle, in practice it was considered useful by less than half the survey respondents. Despite its seemingly widespread use, there was limited support for its role in decision support as it was considered lacking in depth and accuracy. There were a few examples of it being used to identify underfunding in key areas of health and wellbeing, but positive responses were generally limited to it 'showing promise' and raising questions for further investigation. Interviewees also noted that the data were at least a year out of date and real-time data were needed in order to make sound financial decisions; quality of the data was variable and categories needed disaggregating. For example, programme budgeting data were not stratified by age which caused difficulties for joint planning. One interviewee described the problem as follows:

> 'The local authority they can't understand why we don't know what we spend on children's services. At one level we do but at one level we don't because obviously it's in every bit of our contracts. You have to cut it different ways, programme budgeting doesn't help us with that.' (Director of strategic commissioning, site 10)

There were also concerns among a number of interviewees that programme budgeting was categorised in ways which did not reflect the allocation of preventive resources across specific care pathways nor across different programme areas. In general, preventive aspects of programmes were poorly developed. In focusing on prioritisation of investment within the NHS, possibilities for partnership working could be missed.

Some interviewees were using PBMA for strategic development and recognised its importance in looking at the balance across resources and outcomes across a care pathway.

However, others considered it difficult to implement:

> 'No, no one uses programme budgeting and marginal analysis and they should do ... we all know the theory – doing it is difficult... where are the 50 people that have got really good experience of putting it into practice locally that could come along and go to health authorities and say we're going to give you three sessions and show you how to do this, and we're going to use practical methods and routine data and we'll make a difference for you.' (DPH, site 1)

The concept of value for money in preventive services was considered ill defined and it was difficult to compare costs of preventive services as there were so many different models in use across England.

Preventative health spend

Monitoring a shift in investment towards prevention required identification of PHS, although it was emphasised by PCT interviewees that PHS focused on measuring process rather than outcome. While aspects of programme budgeting and allocations through the primary care budget were indicative of PHS, it was seen as difficult, if not impossible, to define or measure given the number of contexts in which preventive care was delivered. It was sometimes equated with growth money which had been allocated to addressing health inequalities or lifestyle interventions, or as spend which was under the control of the public health department or the health improvement team. There were exceptions, however. Some of the case study sites were committed to identifying and tracking PHS and one site had decided to increase the amount spent on prevention by 0.5% each year and decrease the spend on the acute sector by the same percentage. A director of finance explained:

> 'I mean each year we can say that we're spending this extra money on prevention, but when we've done that baseline assessment, we went right down into well how much of the health visitors' time is about prevention ... and we looked in quite some detail about all the different components that we could say was around health prevention ... what we'd like to do is revisit that and say well, using that same criteria, what does it look like now?' (Site 3)

In this site, the concept of PHS was clearly aligned to shifting the balance of spend towards prevention through the use of programme budgeting data.

The national survey showed that around 55% of responding PCTs were trying to calculate PHS, with programme budgeting being the most common method for achieving this. There was an even split between PCTs that said they tracked PHS (41%) and those who did not (40%), while 45% of PCTs claimed they were using PHS as a strategy for increasing investment in health improvement, through targeted interventions for areas such as obesity and cardiovascular disease.

The business case for investing in health and wellbeing

As shown in Table 6.1, interviewees in each of the case study sites emphasised the importance of presenting a business case for longer-term investment for health and wellbeing, but some were concerned that, although there was an evidence base on the effectiveness of public health interventions, there was insufficient evidence on their cost-effectiveness or on the return on investment over the longer-term. The public health evidence base was comparatively underdeveloped and this could work against PCT board approval for new proposals. There was also the view, however, that public health did not hold the monopoly on a poorly developed evidence base but suffered disproportionately from a lack of investment.

Interviewees commented on the difficulties of prioritising longer-term benefits, and considered that economic arguments for public health investment needed further research and development if public health investment was to compete successfully against arguments for increased resources from health care providers. These views were shared across DsPH, practice-based commissioners and PCT board members:

> 'And so I think that the economic argument for the public health investment needs a lot more research and development and a lot more strengthening because it's stacked up against an economic argument that's compelling from the health care providers.'(NED [non-executive director], site 7) (Marks et al., 2011c: 18)

There were difficulties in choosing between different preventive initiatives, as one DPH commented:

> 'You know, should we put all of our money and spend £5 million and get people to go to Weight Watchers and lose weight or should we spend £5 million on people giving up smoking or a combination of what?' (DPH, site 8)

This view was also reflected among practice-based commissioners:

> 'If we had £100,000 of freed resource, for example, there isn't an off-the-shelf use for that cash. Say we'd like to put £100,000 into this particular area of health improvement and we'd like to buy a £100k's worth of that – that isn't available. It's not been thought through or worked up to the point where we could say all right that's what we want to invest in and know that these are the likely outcomes for that as well.' (PBC lead, site 6)

However, in two sites there was confidence that return on investment could be demonstrated:

> 'There's an evidence base for what works but there's not always an evidence base to show what the return on the investment is....That's what I mean about challenging public health to not sit back and go you've got to ring fence funds for us because we're the Cinderella here.... If you don't want to be slashed, prove you don't want to be slashed, do the return on investment work, and when you do it, you can prove there's a business case in there.' (Director of strategy, site 3)

In another site, health economic modelling had provided a useful resource, demonstrating the economic benefits of intervening in the prevention and primary care element of the care pathway. It was argued that public health had developed 'more of a public health economic outlook'. However, it was recognised that the skills required for health economic modelling were lacking and tools for modelling health impact needed further development:

> 'But the economic analysis has been not sophisticated in any sense at all, and it's one area where we feel, I think, and I don't think we're alone in this, we feel quite vulnerable in terms of our capacity to do that kind of analysis. The skills are relatively rare and, you know, being able to do the marginal analysis and cost-benefit ratios and all those sorts of things, value for money, sort of investment stuff, there's some of it that's okay and we can do, but the actual analytical resource is minimal at the moment.' (DPH, site 4)

Some interviewees expressed scepticism about the process as a whole: there was a lack of time to carry out systematic approaches to prioritisation; skills for using prioritisation tools were in short supply; and weighting of criteria was difficult. The result was a lack of transparency and rigour in the prioritisation process:

> 'So I think having tried to create a rational and straightforward and transparent process, when it actually came down to it, it was largely the kind of gut feelings of four executive directors late on a Friday afternoon about what was a good

thing to do and what was not a good thing to do.' (DPH, site 7) (Marks et al., 2013a: 415)

The variety of local approaches being adopted by PCTs was puzzling to some interviewees, especially given the wealth of research on prioritisation and the fact that all PCTs were trying to address similar issues. There were examples of PCTs liaising over how to develop ethical frameworks in order to be able to score proposals and to provide transparency in decision making: agreement over a 'set of ethical commissioning principles' was suggested.

In general, technical issues of measurement or choice of criteria were discussed rather than underpinning values and ethical issues. It was, however, recognised that the process could not be reduced to a technocratic exercise:

> 'We've all agreed there's no science to it. There's no magical tool that's going to give you the answer and say you should do this beyond that. You know, there are a range of factors that you're going to have to take into account from needs and the financial situation and the political situation and where the public is coming from. So it's trying to get a balance of that and looking at how we use, I suppose tools, if you want to regard them as that. It's health inequalities, impact assessment, equality impact assessment, working with the local authority looking at a sort of integrated impact assessment tool, where you take all these parameters in. It doesn't provide you with the answer, but it makes explicit a lot of the issues and implications of what you're planning to do or not planning to do.' (DPH, site 2)

The economic crisis was described as provoking a more radical approach to overall spend: with an emphasis on prevention to save costs and on assessing the effectiveness of all spend rather than changes at the margin.

Lessons from the research for public health in local government

Responsibility for a public health budget was transferred from the NHS to local authorities in April 2013 and they now hold responsibility for promoting the health of their populations and for addressing health inequalities. This has changed the context for priority setting for public health as well as the accountability arrangements for DsPH and public health teams. While NHS commissioners looked across pathways and programmes of care in order to try and 'shift the gravity of spend', local authority commissioners are likely to consider not only the cost-effective deployment of the ring-fenced budget but also how the budget may be used to enhance or catalyse public health informed decision making and initiatives across all local authority directorates. As part of a separate research project on prioritising public health investment in local authorities, the following questions were suggested as relevant for public health commissioners (Marks et al., 2013b: 8).

- Which public health interventions give rise to the greatest return on investment and over which time periods?
- How should return on investment be calculated and which sectors should be included in estimating costs?
- What is the most cost-effective use of resources for the ring-fenced public health budget?
- Which criteria are important when making prioritisation decisions?
- How can the public health budget create added value for preventive activities delivered by other local authority directorates?
- How can the public health budget be deployed to address the wider determinants of health/health inequalities and address the Marmot agenda (Marmot Review, 2010)?
- Which interventions should be prioritised for specific topics?
- Which decision support approaches are best suited for public health investment/disinvestment across sectors?
- Which priority-setting methods are likely to prove most useful for public health decision makers given the resources and skills available?
- Which approaches are likely to be considered appropriate and legitimate by wider stakeholders and the public?
- How can the health benefits (or harms) of interventions in other sectors be maximised (or minimised)?

Through developing commissioning strategies across directorates, local authorities can develop innovative approaches for engaging those who do not access services, for example, and promote healthier local environments through regeneration, leisure, planning and licensing decisions. In some cases, the public health team has been dispersed across directorates to facilitate this local authority-wide approach. Unlike PCTs, local authorities can also draw on extensive knowledge of local communities and established ways of consulting and involving local people in commissioning decisions. While the concept of PHS could be meaningful in the context of monitoring the extent to which the NHS budget focused on prevention or whether any reconfiguration was taking place, the concept is more difficult to operationalise in a local authority context, given that many local authority responsibilities, such as housing, transport or the environment, already have a public health impact.

While a focus on the social determinants of health has been widely welcomed, this could also lead to reduced emphasis on clinical preventive services, or lifestyle management initiatives. In addition, the economic benefits of prevention may be perceived as largely accruing to the NHS. There could also be fewer incentives for NHS commissioners to focus on preventive aspects of care pathways or on rebalancing total spend towards prevention, given that responsibility for many preventive services now rests with local authorities. However, part of the public health responsibility for local government is to provide advice to clinical commissioning groups (CCGs) on prioritisation processes, including programme budgeting (Department of Health, 2011b).

Despite these changes in context, commissioners will still need access to timely public health intelligence through Public Health England and other agencies, and evidence of effectiveness of public health interventions. These will need to inform transparent approaches to priority setting, although, as described earlier, there is likely to be more emphasis on 'commissioning for value' through options appraisal, cost-impact and cost-benefit analysis, showing costs and benefits across the public sector as a whole, rather than focusing on cost-utility analysis through QALYs. Issues such as impact, feasibility and acceptability will be considered in relation to local strategic priorities. Moreover, decisions are taking place in a political context which will influence definitions of evidence and approaches to priority setting. Although demonstrating return on investment for public health interventions was a key issue for the study, social return on investment – where social value is estimated through a consideration of social, economic and environmental costs and benefits – may better reflect the broader remit of local authorities and models for integrating this approach into a commissioning cycle have been developed (Inglis, 2012). This is also likely to influence the deployment of the public health budget. On the other hand, there are risks of the budget, or a proportion of it, simply being used to reduce deficits, with contributions to longer-term public outcomes as a post hoc rationalisation capable of being applied to a range of council services.

While PCTs in the study needed to work in partnership with local authorities to promote health and wellbeing, HWBs are now the route through which local authorities and CCGs will need to build relationships in order to integrate and coordinate preventive services as well as health and social care services. There is also likely to be variation across authorities in their approach to health improvement. In the study, the primary focus for PBC was demand management rather than longer-term preventive initiatives, and this may be reflected in CCG priorities, as expressed through HWBs. Much is expected of HWBs and reforms are at an early stage at the time of writing. However, an early assessment (NHS Confederation, 2012) showed that while there had been a degree of alignment across JSNAs and other community strategies in some HWBs, and there were examples of cross-cutting responsibilities for health and wellbeing for which all cabinet members were responsible, a focus on wider determinants of health appeared underdeveloped. It noted that:

> few boards have enlisted expertise from people with a background in spatial planning, regeneration, housing, culture and leisure, or industry and commerce. Boards will need to ensure that immediate pressures linked to health and social care issues do not prevent them addressing the challenge of how to improve wellbeing. (NHS Confederation, 2012: 5)

This shows that despite the relocation of public health to local authorities, difficulties in 'shifting the gravity of spend' towards prevention may persist and this will be compounded by the dramatic reduction in resources available to local government.

Conclusions

Priority setting is influenced by social values, national and local priorities, public health intelligence and the need to make the best use of available resources. These inform the choice and weighting of criteria used in the different methods for prioritising public health investment. However, the study showed that methods for priority setting were not always suited to addressing equity or longer-term public health investment, data were often inadequate and modelling skills were in short supply. Narrow approaches to the evidence base and decision making did not reflect the need to anticipate public health challenges before they became widespread and more intractable. Disinvestment in existing services was increasingly considered as a prerequisite for public health investment in a period of austerity, but this was proving difficult to achieve.

The study showed that commissioners made relatively little use of the decision support methods available and tools were often locally developed. The analysis of PHS to identify actual spend or monitor any shifts towards prevention across care pathways or the total budget was limited and, as attempts were made to calculate the public health budget to be transferred to local authorities, the variation across PCTs in historical spend on prevention became obvious.

As the public health budget is prioritised within a local authority context, differences in the approaches to prioritisation are likely to emerge. A tradition of options appraisal, value for money and demonstrating social return on investment in a context of democratic accountability lends itself to a more participative and intersectoral approach to commissioning and priority setting, although, as for PCTs in the study, relevant health economic and modelling skills remain in short supply. With economic pressures and deficits facing local authorities, developing frameworks for prioritisation will become increasingly urgent if transparency in making difficult rationing decisions is to be achieved.

Notes

[1] See: http://guidance.nice.org.uk/PHG/Published.

[2] See: www.who.int/topics/global_burden_of_disease/en/

[3] See: www.scenario-generator.com/.

[4] See: www.apho.org.uk/resource/item.aspx?RID=100181.

[5] Available at: www.apho.org.uk/resource/item.aspx?RID=78141.

CHAPTER SEVEN

Public involvement in commissioning

> 'What I'm saying is, it's about levels of governance. Our aspiration, I hope, is that we have some kind of accountability to local people, but actually if we're really going to make that real, we have a huge piece of work on our hands.' (National focus group)

As described in Chapter Two, participation and accountability are intrinsic to governance. This chapter is concerned with aspects of public accountability, in particular, ways of engaging and representing the public in commissioning decisions, and the role of local authority overview and scrutiny committees (OSCs), which had been set up to strengthen public accountability. Public involvement in commissioning is intended to promote transparency in decision making and is also seen as a route for ensuring that services are relevant to people's needs. It is argued that involving local communities in commissioning can also help ensure effective implementation of health promotion strategies and is more likely to result in the effective mobilising of community assets and the engagement of local community organisations. However, as originally reflected in Arnstein's eight-step ladder of engagement (Arnstein, 1969) there is a spectrum of involvement, culminating with citizen control – a concept which applies to individual consumers as well as to the public as collective decision makers (Harrison et al., 2002).

Involvement in decisions about individual treatment and care, or about the quality of services, forms only part of the picture and is not to be equated with broader public involvement in decisions over the nature, accessibility and prioritisation of services related to health and the prevention of ill health. The two areas are not mutually exclusive: as one example, involvement of patients and expert patient groups in redesigning pathways of care for specific conditions is a well-established route for informing commissioning decisions. However, public involvement in commissioning raises broader governance issues related to accountability and representation. Although it has its own history and dynamic, patient and public involvement in health (PPI) does not occur in isolation from wider political and policy commitments to promote public participation, scrutiny and community engagement in decision making. The importance of community-based and participative approaches in developing social capital and addressing health inequalities is increasingly recognised in national and international policy initiatives and reiterated in *Health 2020* (WHO, 2012a). While this chapter focuses on public involvement in commissioning, rather than on patient involvement in treatment and care, underserved groups are unlikely to become engaged in either without concurrent initiatives for asset-based approaches to capacity building (Foot and Hopkins, 2010) and participatory approaches to community development (Springett, 2001). The importance of public engagement has also been highlighted from an economic perspective. It was considered a key aspect of the 'fully engaged' scenario described in the Wanless reports (Wanless, 2002, 2004), where not just the health of the population but also the future sustainability of the NHS was considered to depend on 'fully engaged' citizens, in the light of the increasing economic burden from non-communicable diseases. However, progress was slow, as underlined in an update to the Wanless report which stated (Wanless et al., 2007: 181):

> The evidence rules out a fully engaged scenario of public engagement in improving the determinants of health. Public engagement falls somewhere between solid progress and slow uptake.

This chapter begins by discussing participatory governance and outlines parameters of patient and public involvement, including changes introduced during the period of the Labour government. Drawing on the study, it describes initiatives for public involvement in commissioning for health and wellbeing and how they were viewed in practice. As described in Chapter Three, over the period of the study the commissioning role of primary care trusts (PCTs) had become more clearly defined and separated from the provision of services. This raised the question of how best to reflect local views in the commissioning cycle, as well as in the better established area of patient and public involvement in treatment and care.

Participatory governance

> How to create flexible and effective organisations for delivering public services that also reflect the values of

local democracy. We call this 'citizen-centred' governance.
(Barnes et al., 2008: 1)

The commitment of the main political parties to devolving power to local democratic structures, users and local communities reflects the importance of improving accountability and encouraging 'active citizenship'. A variety of terms, such as 'community governance', 'neighbourhood governance', 'citizen-centred governance', 'co-governance' or 'participatory (local) governance' reflects these values of democratic accountability and of public involvement. Community participation forms part of 'good governance' and is seen as a source of social capital and considered of intrinsic value (Osmani, 2008). The development of formal structures for user involvement across public services therefore reflects the importance attached to civic participation in governance and scrutiny of these services. The 2011 Localism Bill, introduced by the coalition government, was intended to 'empower communities to do things their way' (HM Government, 2010b), with a 'radical shift' of power from the centralised state to local communities and neighbourhood governance. In practice, potential freedoms were overshadowed by financial austerity and there are disagreements over how civil society and 'community' are to be defined, and the extent to which a shift in meaningful engagement is being achieved in practice. Jochum et al. (2005) had argued that there is often a gap between the rhetoric and the reality of engagement, that 'the devolution of power that would lead to meaningful engagement is not taking place', and that managerial approaches to involvement are becoming widespread as the third sector professionalises. These arguments are reflected in more recent debates over 'the Big Society', where the rhetoric of involvement has been undermined by the reality of a decline in funding for local community organisations.

While a localism agenda is intended to help shift the balance from 'government' to 'governance', Barnes et al. (2008) described a 'patchwork of governance arrangements', arising from a plethora of statutory agencies, partnerships and boards. The complexity of these overlapping structures resulted in a proliferation of mapping exercises attempting to capture local arrangements, local governance structures and their impact on engagement, as well as qualitative research on the experience of engagement within certain neighbourhoods and groups (Maguire and Truscott, 2006; Marks, 2007). At a local level, the mix of governance arrangements can lead to consultation overlap and confused accountability.

Routes for engagement in commissioning include local authority democratic structures; health and wellbeing boards (HWBs) and their constituent organisations, including local Healthwatch; and voluntary and community sector (VCS) membership of partnership boards. Clinical commissioning groups (CCGs) have a duty to involve the public in commissioning decisions and were required to demonstrate 'meaningful engagement with patients, carers and their communities' as part of the authorisation process (Department of Health, 2011c). CCG governing bodies also have a local lay member. Other common routes for patient and public engagement in the NHS include patient participation groups, citizens' juries, focus groups and public meetings and there is scope for CCGs, for example, to develop a range of approaches (NHS Confederation, 2011b). Also intended to strengthen public accountability are local authority OSCs for health, set up in 2003 to scrutinise health services and health issues and identify areas of concern to the public. In each local area, there is also a wide range of voluntary and community organisations, often formed into local networks and playing an important role in partnership organisations (such as local strategic partnerships [LSPs] prior to April 2013 and HWBs thereafter), regeneration partnerships and locality or neighbourhood arrangements. There are, therefore, complex patterns of public involvement and routes for engagement across the local authority, the local NHS, the VCS and localities.

Despite this emphasis on public involvement, the drive for greater efficiency creates services which cover larger geographical areas, remote from local decision making. These issues are of relevance for commissioners as they have a duty to engage with local populations. Moreover, many governance structures are not suited to community engagement. A mix of governance arrangements can lead to consultation overlap, confused accountability and lack of clarity over representation. Barnes et al. (2008) also corroborate findings of previous research regarding uncertainties over whether community participation is based on local knowledge or the ability to represent particular groups or areas and, in the case of the latter, whether there are clear mechanisms for ensuring representation. Moreover, 'newer' forms of governance may lack formal legal status, and show lower levels of transparency and accountability to the public than statutory bodies.

Patient and public involvement in context

Patient and public involvement in health has taken a number of different forms, leading to a plethora of different initiatives, organisations and routes for encouraging involvement which, in turn, take their cue from the multiple expectations associated with the role. These include, in various permutations: involving patients in treatment and care options; incorporating patient and carer views on the quality of local services; providing channels for feedback on services and for complaints; involving local groups in identifying health needs in their local community and in underserved groups; addressing the lack of democratic accountability in the NHS through greater collective involvement in decision making; and representing local communities in the commissioning cycle. While public involvement in commissioning draws on a well-established tradition of PPI in health care, it is also informed by this wider range of (sometimes conflicting) routes for local involvement. The context and development of PPI in health care is described before discussing involvement in commissioning practice and the shift to democratic accountability for public health commissioning.

Policy background: from community health councils to Healthwatch

As illustrated in Box 7.1, PPI has taken many different forms and is often reshaped in the context of NHS reorganisation. Community health councils (CHCs) were set up in 1974, with the intention of giving patients and the public a voice in the NHS. The confusing trajectory and varying roles of PPI from the demise of CHCs in 2003 to the current configuration of national and local Healthwatch is, perhaps, a reflection of multiple expectations. The tendency to conflate patient and user involvement in treatment or health care services with collective public involvement in decision making, combined with ambiguity about their purpose, has led to what has been described as 'muddled initiatives and uncertainty about what should be done to achieve effective patient and public involvement' (House of Commons Health Committee, 2007: 3).

Box 7.1: Patient and public involvement: organisational structures

1974: Community health councils (CHCs), with elected members, were established in England and Wales. There was a duty to consult CHCs over 'substantial developments or variations' to health services.

2000: The 'Expert Patients' initiative was included in the NHS Plan (2000) and helped support the notion of co-creation of services.

2001: Overview and scrutiny committees (OSCs), with elected local authority councillors were established. Their remit was extended to health in 2003 and intended to promote accountability in health services.

2003: CHCs in England were replaced by the combination of patient and public involvement forums (PPIFs), the Patient Advice and Liaison Service (PALS) and the Independent Complaints Advocacy Service (ICAS).

2003: PPIFs were established and supported by a national Commission for Patient and Public Involvement in Health. Over 550 PPIFs were initially set up (one for every NHS Trust and PCT in England).

2003: A PALS was established in every healthcare trust while the ICAS covered formal complaints.

2004: Foundation Trusts (FTs) were intended to promote a level of community ownership through elected lay governors. FTs are accountable to their members.

2004: The Healthcare Commission was set up under the Health and Social Care (Community Health and Standards) Act 2003.

2007: Local involvement networks (LINks) were established through the Labour government's Local Government and Public Involvement in Health Bill. LINks were based in each local authority area with a social services responsibility, comprised individuals and community groups and spanned health and social care across a local authority area. No national LINks organisation was set up at the time, although support was available from the NHS Centre for Involvement (disbanded in 2009).

2008: PPIFs and the National Commission for Patient and Public Involvement in Health were abolished.

2009: The Care Quality Commission replaced the Healthcare Commission, the Commission for Social Care Inspection and the Mental Health Act Commission.

2013: Local Healthwatch and Healthwatch England were established through the Health and Social Care Act 2012, and were intended to replace LINks. Local Healthwatch is located in each local authority area and is a core member of the statutory health and wellbeing board. Healthwatch England is a statutory committee of the Care Quality Commission with an advisory role to the Department of Health as well as to NHS England.

The former Labour government promoted numerous initiatives for encouraging public involvement in decision making, and the duties of providers and commissioners to involve and consult were made more explicit. This priority was reflected in policy, legislation, standard setting, monitoring and performance management arrangements, and was also included in commissioning competencies for PCTs. LINks (local involvement networks) were implemented from 2008 to promote greater public involvement in health and social care.

Greater public involvement was reflected in the Local Government Act 2000, which placed a duty on local authorities to engage local communities in decision making and introduced the scrutiny function into local government. Subsequently, *Strong and prosperous communities: The local government White Paper* (Secretary of State for Communities and Local Government, 2006) called for 'more visible local leadership for health and wellbeing', partnerships and joined-up performance management approaches, and 'greater clarity' over agreeing and delivering local health and wellbeing targets. To this end, statutory health and wellbeing partnership boards were proposed, although they were not enshrined in legislation in the ensuing Local Government and Public Involvement in Health Act 2007. They were, however, revived in the coalition government's White Paper, *Equity and excellence: Liberating the NHS* (Secretary of State for Health, 2010a: para. 4.17) and implemented in each upper-tier and unitary authority from April 2013.

The Health and Social Care Act 2001 (Section 11) and subsequently the NHS Act 2006 (Section 242) had also provided for extensive public consultation and involvement in developing, planning and delivery of health services. The latter provided for a legal 'duty to involve' patients and their representatives in the planning and provision of services and over proposed changes to statutory NHS services. The White Paper *Our health, our care, our say* (Secretary of State for Health, 2006) called for 'more choice and a louder voice' and included the aims of a stronger user and citizen role in commissioning, in improving services, in assessing service quality and in regulation, and in holding the system to account. This led to a review of patient and public involvement, culminating in *A stronger local voice*, which elaborated how people could have more say in how the health and social care system was designed (Department of Health, 2006b). At the time of the study, the *Commissioning framework for health and well-being* (Department of Health, 2007a) recommended that commissioners should 'empower everyone to be able to make choices that promote their health and wellbeing' ('choice') (p. 21), as well as enabling people to exercise 'greater voice and influence'. The latter was to be achieved through public and user involvement in commissioning, priority setting and service development: commissioners could draw on various methods for community engagement, as well as on the activities of LINks, set up with the specific purpose of promoting local involvement and gathering local views of health and social services (p. 22).

Involvement was further elaborated through *Real involvement: Working with people to improve health services* (Department of Health, 2008d), which outlined principles for local accountability and provided guidance for the NHS on the duty to involve. A spectrum of involvement was outlined, including involvement in commissioning decisions across the commissioning cycle, in practice-based commissioning (PBC) and representation in governance structures (p. 28). Also in 2008, the White Paper *Communities in control: Real people, real power* (Secretary of State for Communities and Local Government, 2008) described ways in which people could exert more influence in decision making.

This emphasis on involvement was not only reflected in the remit of new organisations but had also been enshrined in a standard-based planning framework for health and social care (Department of Health, 2004). Standards for health care, used by the former Healthcare Commission as the basis of their annual health check for NHS organisations, included patient and public involvement in designing, planning and delivering services as a core standard. The Healthcare Commission was replaced by the Care Quality Commission (CQC) and the coalition government subsequently replaced the annual health check with registration requirements with a narrower remit, focused on patient involvement and standards of service providers.

The principle of involvement was finally enshrined in the NHS Constitution (Department of Health, 2013b: 3), which stated that 'patients, with their families and carers, where appropriate, will be involved in and consulted on all decisions about their care and treatment'. A statement of NHS accountability (Department of Health, 2009d), which accompanied the original NHS Constitution in 2010, took a broader approach, expanding on four main ways that local accountability could be achieved, namely: the duty to involve and report to the public; Foundation Trust membership; independent LINks; and local authority OSCs (comprised of elected councillors and supported by council officials). There was, therefore, no doubt about the policy priority attached to increasing public involvement.

The coalition government emphasised individual patient choice and adopted the slogan of the patient movement of 'no decisions about me without me' in the NHS White Paper, *Equity and excellence* (Secretary of State for Health, 2010a). The Health and Social Care Act 2012 aimed to increase democratic accountability and legitimacy through the relocation of public health commissioning into local authorities, with additional responsibilities over and above their existing remit to promote 'social, economic and environmental wellbeing'. It aimed to increase the influence of patients through promoting choice and through a new national organisation, Healthwatch England, a statutory committee of the CQC (although operationally independent) and intended to support 152 local Healthwatch organisations across England. New HWBs provided a new forum for decision making related to health and for the production of joint health and wellbeing strategies designed to inform commissioning decisions.

Public involvement through LINks and scrutiny

The Local Government and Public Involvement in Health Act 2007 provided for the abolition of patient and public involvement forums (PPIFs) and the creation of LINks. Their remit included promoting public involvement in the commissioning, provision and scrutiny of health and social services, and obtaining the views of local people. At the time of the study, therefore, LINks were the organisations specifically set up to reflect the views of patients and the public in relation to health and social care. Unlike the former PPIFs, they were not based around particular organisations (that is, PCTs and NHS Trusts) but across a local authority area, thereby better reflecting local communities. They were intended to improve local accountability and reflect all sectors of the community, including user groups, the VCS, Foundation Trust members and neighbourhood groups, as well as individuals. They provided an additional (but not the sole) mechanism for consultation and for making the views of local people known to local commissioners, providers and regulators. Accountable to the public (through publishing an annual report of their activities), LINks reported directly to the Secretary of State for Health. Operating independently from the local authority, they had their own governance structures and decision-making processes. However, they were financially supported by local authorities, which were obliged to set up a 'host' to support the new organisations. Their role was to 'encourage and support local people to get involved in how local care services are planned and run' (Department of Health, 2008e: 2). LINks had the right under the 2007 Act to obtain replies to requests for information, to enter and view specific health and social care premises, and to refer issues to OSC Health Scrutiny Panels. PCTs had to respond to reports and recommendations made through LINks: their role in commissioning was therefore made clear at the outset and they were intended to help commissioners make informed decisions as well as provide feedback to service providers.

Local authority-based OSCs were also intended to strengthen public accountability and their remit was extended to health (in January 2003), although focus groups in the study commented that OSCs were typically focused on the health care system and did not reflect the wider public health agenda. OSCs could also identify issues of concern to the public and were encouraged to focus on the work of commissioners. Supported by the Centre for Public Scrutiny, they were intended to combine broad health promotion functions with the more familiar health service monitoring role (Campbell and Heron, 2010). Guidance (Department of Health, 2003b: 6) noted that:

> The Government's intention is that the focus of health scrutiny is on health improvement, bringing together the responsibilities of local authorities to promote social, environmental and economic wellbeing and the power to scrutinise local services provided and commissioned by the NHS.

The Statement of NHS Accountability (Department of Health, 2009d) further described their role as requiring the NHS to provide information about how local health needs were being addressed. They could co-opt members of the public and were intended to liaise with LINks (and subsequently with local Healthwatch). In their review of OSCs from 2002 to 2005, Coleman and Harrison (2006: 8) note that implementation of the scrutiny role in primary health care was varied, pointing to a 'lack of clarity in both local authorities and the NHS over the relationship between health scrutiny and the wider patient/public policy agenda'. This lack of clarity over the role and purpose of PPI and the resources required to fulfil these roles effectively was reflected in a House of Commons Health Committee report (2007) on the topic of PPI. The Health Committee noted that the concept of LINks had changed over time from 'a network to aid consultation' to a 'PPIF plus model', which would involve volunteers undertaking a similar range of activities to those formerly carried out by PPIFs, but with the addition of greater involvement in commissioning. However, a network model could prove time consuming and difficult to achieve within allocated resources. Moreover, while experienced volunteers could be lost in the transition from PPIFs to LINks, a wholesale transfer from one organisation to the other could make it difficult to change perspectives in line with new responsibilities and exacerbate a focus on health rather than on health and social care. The Committee raised questions over the role of LINks, including their overlap with local authority and other monitoring bodies, and recommended that fundamental questions should be addressed, such as their remit and level of independence, membership, funding, focus and national coordination. Nevertheless, membership, organisation and accountability arrangements were all left vague and the balance to be struck between engagement with, or co-option by, commissioners remained unresolved. While a less prescriptive approach was a deliberate attempt to move away from what had come to be seen as an over-prescriptive and centralised model of patient forums, this also led to differing assumptions and expectations at a local level about roles and responsibilities of LINks (Melvin, 2010).

From LINks to Healthwatch

Local Healthwatch, established from April 2013, and commissioned by local authorities, were designed to be independent organisations taking over the statutory functions of LINks, as well as additional responsibilities. They are required to provide information about local care services and choices to be made in respect of those services to service users and to provide feedback to Healthwatch England (and, if necessary, the CQC) about the quality of services (Local Government Association, 2013). Unlike LINks, their remit includes capturing the voice of children and young people in relation to health and social care services and local Healthwatch is a core member of statutory HWBs. While much of the policy emphasis is on patient involvement in care and treatment, and on choice of healthcare providers, Healthwatch England is developing its role as a 'consumer champion' within a framework of consumer rights, drawing on international guidelines for consumer protection and in consultation with local Healthwatch representatives. It has put forward eight consumer rights for health and social care (Healthwatch England, 2013). One of these rights is the 'right to be involved', not just in care but, as a citizen, in decisions about health and social care services. Another right is to 'live in an environment that promotes health and wellbeing'. There is, therefore, a sustained policy emphasis on greater involvement and accountability. Whether local governance has been achieved in practice, however, is open to question.

This brief overview illustrates the expectations of the new PPI organisations at the time of the study, how they differed from previous PPI initiatives through their closer relationship with local authorities and with local government scrutiny functions, and how the role has been developed through local Healthwatch. Although the study predates local Healthwatch and the reorganisation of commissioning, themes of representativeness, governance and accountability are likely to persist in the new arrangements.

Public involvement in practice

The introduction of world class commissioning (WCC), in 2007, provided the means for integrating greater public involvement into the commissioning cycle. The *Commissioning framework for health and well-being* (Department of Health, 2007a), which foreshadowed WCC, had described people as lying 'at the centre of commissioning' – noting that 'the challenge to commissioners is how to make greater local voice, choice and control a reality' (para. 2.1). Commissioners were encouraged to develop 'mechanisms for patients and service users, as well as the general public, to get involved in shaping commissioning priorities and services' (para. 2.4). The WCC 'vision' (Department of Health, 2007b: 3) was non-negotiable in its demands for public involvement in commissioning, stating that:

> World Class Commissioners will engage with the public, and actively seek the views of patients, carers and the wider community. This new relationship with the public is long-term, inclusive and enduring and has been forged through a sustained effort and commitment on the part of commissioners. Decisions are made with a strong mandate from the local population and other partners.

The role of PPI in commissioning decisions was reflected in the WCC assurance handbook, in related guidance and in performance management arrangements. While the coalition government abolished the infrastructure of performance management reflected in WCC, the emphasis on patient and public involvement remained.

This section reviews routes for public involvement in commissioning and for involvement of the public in aspects of the commissioning cycle and in PBC, based on study findings. Roles in decision making and scrutiny are illustrated through views of three different groups: VCS members of health and wellbeing subgroups of LSPs; Chairs of LINks; and Chairs of health scrutiny committees of the OSC, who are elected local councillors. Box 7.2 outlines the research methods adopted for this aspect of the study.

Box 7.2 Public involvement in commissioning: study methods

The study involved an in-depth analysis of 10 case study sites across England and out of a total number of 99 interviews (carried out over two phases) 25 were carried out with members of the public, namely health scrutiny committee chairs (6), LINk chairs (9) and VCS members of partnerships (10). All interviewees, including chief executives, directors of finance, commissioning and public health, PBC leads and non-executive directors (NEDs) were asked how the public was currently involved in commissioning. The study also carried out a national survey to provide a context for local findings and three focus groups, which also discussed public involvement in commissioning.

While PCT interviewees in the study drew attention to a wide range of initiatives to involve the public, the VCS and LINks in commissioning and decision making, in many cases PPI was described as needing development, especially in areas where the local VCS was not well organised or had been cut back. Initiatives from the 10 case study sites are summarised in Box 7.3, although there was variation between sites in the degree and intensity of engagement. There was also engagement through the local VCS organisations and the influence of LINks was generally viewed by PCTs as only part of a wide spectrum of patient and public involvement.

Box 7.3: Methods for encouraging public involvement in commissioning

A wide variety of methods were used in the study to engage with local communities:

- public and patient engagement strategies, sometimes developed in conjunction with local authorities and the VCS;
- public involvement in the JSNA (joint strategic needs assessment) was encouraged through a range of methods, including large consultative exercises, leaflet drops and media campaigns;
- LINks representatives could be included on JSNA steering groups;
- public involvement in strategic commissioning forums;
- large stakeholder events to inform strategy;
- focus groups, patient panels and citizens' panels;
- 'health' conversations;
- telephone surveys;
- prioritisation initiatives, including community conferences, prioritisation workshops and public strategic commissioning forums;

- the payment of sessional fees to members of the public to encourage engagement;
- involvement of the public in assessing bids;
- developing networks for patients to become involved in service redesign, pathway work and service specifications, and patient and public involvement in each programme area;
- population profiling, such as through Mosaic and social marketing, to identify better ways of engaging with specific populations which in turn could influence commissioning strategy;
- lay representatives on subcommittees of the PCT board or on the board itself as non-voting members;
- open sessions with the public prior to PCT board meetings;
- patient advisory forums which were representative of the population;
- locality-based approaches bringing together service providers, councillors and residents and feeding into Borough-wide partnership boards.

In one of the sites, where the PCT was considered proactive in engaging with the VCS, there had been a year-long and widely publicised exercise to engage the public in the principles and criteria for investment. Practice-based commissioners had also started to hold public meetings over their plans. In another site, nominated LINk members were involved in working groups, tender panels, specifications and pathway redesign. A further site held 15 community conferences across the most disadvantaged 30% of the population, in order to get a community voice in commissioning decisions.

There were also examples of joint strategies with local authorities, including locality forums, to avoid inundating the public with requests for information, described as follows:

> 'Sometimes we're trying to both reach the same people but doing it separately. So I think joining up some of the resources we have and the engagement mechanisms, we've got some that are already joint but doing more of that I think would be very helpful.' (Director of strategic commissioning, site 10)

These findings were reflected in responses to the national survey, where PCT respondents were asked about mechanisms for public involvement in decision making. Seventy PCTs responded (with a total of 101 responses). Respondents could select as many choices as applicable to their PCT. The results are illustrated in Figure 7.1.

Figure 7.1: Involving local people

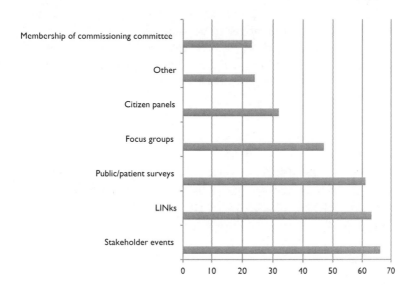

Source: (Marks et al., 2011a: 76)

The survey also sought examples of where local people or groups had influenced commissioning for health and wellbeing services. There were more than 70 responses, with most falling into the following categories: consultation as part of the joint strategic needs assessment (JSNA) process (focus groups and surveys); consultation as part of formulating commissioning strategy plans (for example, 'visioning events'); input into service (re)design (such as for sexual health or mental health services); consultation as part of prioritisation processes; and focus groups used in developing social marketing. Participants in focus groups carried out as part of the study also emphasised the use of social marketing to develop and target messages. This could include the involvement of the VCS and working through social networks.

A number of themes relating to public involvement were shared across PCT interviewees. First was the difficulty of engaging the public, with a number of interviewees commenting on the importance of avoiding over-representation of 'single issue' groups or 'monopolisation' of the agenda by certain sectors of the VCS. Even where there was a well-organised VCS network or consortium, the range and diversity of organisations could make it difficult for them to liaise and to reflect views.

Second was the difficulty of achieving representation from different cultural groups, from disadvantaged or transient populations and areas where there was a high turnover in population.

Third was a relative lack of interest in preventive services which meant that public involvement was skewed towards health care services. This was cited in eight of the ten case study sites. One interviewee commented:

> 'I keep saying this to loads of people, very boringly, that most people, you know, if they're not ill, are not really focused on health. What they're focused on is have they got enough money to live, you know, is their house in good condition, you know, is there poverty around and all sorts of other things that absolutely are determinants of ill health, but they're the most important things in people's heads.' (Deputy chief executive, site 8)

Public health services lacked visibility, received less public and media attention, and were described as low on the public's 'worry list'.

> 'It's not unique to the UK, most countries have this problem, and that's because the public can see health care. They can see health care, for some reason, but they can't see health; health is pretty much invisible.' (Non-executive director, site 7)

Fourth were issues of access and engagement. Some PCT interviewees argued that there were few natural points of contact for engaging the public in a health and wellbeing agenda, as opposed to a health care agenda, and that it was often people who had been ill who were involved in order that their perspective and experience informed the commissioning process.

Rather different views were expressed by VCS interviewees. They focused on the importance of locally relevant issues, of demonstrating the impact of public involvement on decision making and clarifying the levels at which the public could be involved – from the strategic level to more detailed pathway redesign or service development. The role of the VCS was crucial in reaching disadvantaged groups and this needed to be taken into account in commissioning decisions, avoiding dangers of professionalising the third sector 'so that they're not of and by the communities any more'. If this was not taken into consideration, there was a danger that the ability to engage with disadvantaged groups would be lost.

It was important to develop better flows of information between commissioners and the public, avoid bureaucratic structures which discouraged engagement and for the public to be involved early in the decision-making process. Despite policy priorities for a stronger voice for local communities in commissioning, focus group participants argued that, in practice, local engagement in decision making was minimal and there was little local accountability. While the process for prioritising was likely to become more transparent with increasing public involvement, tensions would remain between achieving economies of scale offered by large commissioning organisations at the same time as encouraging local involvement. These tensions were inherent in the commissioning process and compounded by a lack of clarity over roles and responsibilities, further described below.

Roles and responsibilities of LINks

LINks were in place in seven of the case study sites when the study began. They saw their role as developing networks and engaging at grassroots level, taking the views of local people to commissioners and vice versa, and challenging commissioners to achieve the best possible services for local populations. In one site, for example, the LINk was developing a stakeholder group with representation from the PCT, the local authority and additional partners. LINks engaged with the public in various ways, including websites, stakeholder events, open board meetings and communication through the local VCS. The partnership and membership within LINks, particularly of the VCS, was seen as a useful way to cascade and disseminate information to a variety of organisations. However, LINks faced a number of challenges common to public involvement strategies, in particular, achieving representative membership. This echoes some of the concerns of PCT interviewees, mentioned earlier:

> 'But I do think that LINks has got to make sure that it doesn't become ... the "usual suspects" syndrome where you just turn out the same people all the time. There's nothing that makes you less credible than that, and LINks has got to make sure that doesn't happen.' (LINk chair, site 3)

There was some concern over insufficient resources and time to fulfil duties, lack of support from the hosts and lack of a campaign to publicise their existence. It was also more difficult to engage with social care than with health services.

Most interviewees felt that it was too early to influence formal decision-making bodies across the local area, as LINks were still forming relationships. Most had little or no input into targets or priority setting, although there was some 'informal acknowledgement' by PCTs of their views. Some considered that LINks had achieved less engagement than the PPIFs which preceded them, although it was difficult to measure public engagement in commissioning or assess influence:

> 'I think it's a difficult thing to do because there are various strands to it and not all easily understandable and you can be involved in something like being consulted on some service or some change in service without realising that you're actually being involved in commissioning, and I think there's quite a lot of that going on.' (LINk chair, site 7)

PCTs were often perceived as commissioning according to a preconceived agenda and it was argued that greater clarity was needed over the role of LINks within statutory organisations:

> 'It still sort of feels as though it's very much like yes we're really interested in what you think about what we're doing, rather than "What should we be doing?".' (LINk chair, site 7)

Some interviewees commented on the lack of interest or engagement from the public. This meant that recruitment to LINk management boards had proved difficult which, in turn, raised questions about their sustainability. However, one site stood out as having a very active LINk that had influenced PCT contract specification. The chair was a co-opted member on the scrutiny panel, a non-voting member on the PCT board and the local LINk was represented on the PBC group, provider organisations, various task groups and committees, and on the local health and wellbeing committee. The organisation had built on aspects of the former PPIF including a panel, now extended to encompass both health and social care, with members available for surveys, or to act as representatives. The panel had good representation from minority groups and held an annual showcase of relevant organisations. They had set up a database of organisations and negotiated training for lay members of committees. Governance arrangements were being developed which would include an annual citizens meeting and there were also plans to bring together patient participation groups based in GP practices to help coordinate views. There was extensive membership with around 600 individual members and 200 organisations, described as follows:

> 'So, for example, LINk works on the premise that anybody can be a member of LINk, whatever member means, and our job is to make sure that we are continually giving them information about what's happening in the health and social care world.... it's no good a group of clinicians and administrators sitting in the PCT working out what specification it ought to be, because they get some disasters. They've got to be out there in the community and in my opinion they have to use LINk to do it.' (LINk chair, site 3)

In this case, a clear distinction was made between the PPIF, the voice of the patient and the LINk, the 'facilitator of the voice' with its connection to the community:

> 'That's really crucial, because once you start moving back to be the patient voice, you're no different from the old PPI forum, which was a patient voice, and if you move back there, your connection with the community weakens all the time because you're not going to the community and saying what do you think, you know, how does this work ... to me that's a really key feature of LINk.' (LINk chair, site 3)

Although LINks had connections with OSCs, as anticipated in the guidance, they were yet to form strong relationships with partnership organisations, such as LSPs, or with practice-based commissioners, many of whom seemed unaware of the existence of LINks at the time of the interviews. It was argued that the structure of local partnerships and LINks' place within them needed to be to be clarified, and that there should also be clear routes through which LINks could influence social care.

The majority of PCT interviewees acknowledged LINks' potential as a source of information and as a gateway to a more systematic engagement with the VCS. In one site, the LINk was integrated into the JSNA process as well as into commissioning subcommittees of the PCT board, and in two sites LINks had a seat on the PCT board. However, many PCT interviewees were unclear to what extent patient representatives might also be members of LINks, which were generally viewed as forming only a part of wider engagement strategies. One interviewee considered that they reflected a 'diffuse series of constituencies', and were not a suitable proxy for patient and public engagement. The latter was of a higher priority than involving LINks per se:

> 'It doesn't matter to me, do you know what I mean? As long as I've got members of the public engaged in it, in terms of looking at what we're going to do.' (Director of quality, site 9)

In both phases of interviews, relationships between LINks and umbrella bodies for local voluntary organisations were described as a source of tension, due to overlapping networks and some duplication of roles. The study demonstrated wide variation in the development of LINks as well as in engagement with them, and this variation was more marked than for any other aspect of the study.

Public involvement in the commissioning cycle

As mentioned earlier, public involvement in the commissioning cycle gained greater prominence at the time of the study. WCC required such involvement (Department of Health, 2007c) expressed through competency two (work collaboratively with community partners to commission services that optimise health gains and reductions in health inequalities) and competency three (to proactively seek and build continuous and meaningful engagement with the public and patients, to shape services and improve health). Involvement was intended to mirror the commissioning cycle from assessment of health needs to prioritising investment (or disinvestment) (Department of Health, 2008a). In practice, this could be reflected through formal membership or involvement of the VCS or LINks in decision-making bodies, such as LSPs and their various subgroups; PBC consortia; or PCT boards or their various subcommittees. Whether the rhetoric of engagement was reflected in practice was explored through the study.

Involvement in the JSNA (described in Chapter Three) seemed limited in the case study sites. Only one of the LINk interviewees had been involved in developing the JSNA. However, there were attempts to engage with the public, using a variety of consultation methods. The national survey showed that consultation as part of the JSNA process (focus groups and surveys) was the most widespread activity. It is possible, however, that involvement in participation events was not always formally linked to the JSNA.

Two VCS interviewees stated that public involvement and engagement had been a largely 'tick box' exercise:

> 'It doesn't really happen, well not in commissioning. I mean everybody talks about commissioning. I think it's very hard to see the direct relationship between local people's input and how that's actually influenced the commissioning decisions.' (VCS member, site 4)

The impact of involvement needed to be clarified, with better channels of communication between commissioners and the public:

> 'I mean I think people are more likely to become involved in activities if they think they're making a difference, and I think what has happened in some cases in the past has been where people have come along to consultation events, they've given their views, they've taken the time to do that, and they never know what has happened to them, or they think perhaps they've been ignored.' (VCS member, site 10)

Involving the VCS had been made more complex due to competitive tendering and changes in procurement guidance. The combination of commissioning and provider roles could also create conflicts of interest. In one site, some VCS groups had been excluded from the JSNA due to potential conflicts of interest as they were also involved in providing services. It was argued that one of the drawbacks of WCC was that it was geared to major providers and this made it difficult to contract with the VCS, even though they were in touch with those least likely to engage with services. A number of interviewees commented on the need to take a more radical approach to commissioning preventive services, drawing on new ways of working from the VCS. One interviewee commented:

> 'Instead they're giving the contracts to the big nationals and those nationals haven't got the local social capital, the local sign-up, the localism.' (VCS member, site 9)

Public involvement in practice-based commissioning

In most sites, public involvement in PBC was described as 'developing'. Examples included the public being invited to attend consultations on PBC plans and PBC developing links with local groups around specific conditions. There was sometimes representation on local PBC executive boards and public involvement could be incentivised through a LES (local enhanced service; see Chapter Five) and could contribute to pathway redesign. In two sites, however, PBC consortia had wide membership, including social services and representatives of the public. In one of these sites, there was public involvement not only at practice level but also within locality based partnerships. In other cases, public involvement at PBC level was poorly developed, with a PBC lead commenting:

> 'The other gap I think in terms of practice-based commissioning is that there isn't much direct patient or public involvement in it either, so perhaps we're not seeing things from that perspective as much as we could do.' (Site 6)

Even where there was apparent involvement, a PBC lead stated that public views were insufficiently represented:

> 'I mean every practice has a public involvement group, and the practices are represented by the elected members, and the elected members sit on the executive. You know, from that point of view you could say we are represented.... But it's, again a lot of the meetings we talk in medical jargon, and it's quite strange for somebody sitting in on a meeting.' (Site 5)

Focus group participants also considered engagement to be minimal:

> 'On the whole it's an underlying paternalistic culture within primary care, an assumption by GPs and perhaps practice nurses and some practice staff, that they are in the best position to know what members of their patient list want and not, and be unwilling or unable to see the benefits of asking the people that they serve what they would like.' (National focus group)

With the exception of one site, PBC interviewees had not heard of LINks. A few interviewees were sceptical about the benefits of public involvement in decision making. However, as discussed further below, representatives from the VCS and LINks felt they could and should influence commissioning strategies. Their involvement could improve accountability to the public, as they could both gather and disseminate relevant information through their members and through local networks.

Influencing decision making through partnerships

A capacity to engage effectively with the VCS was identified as a key factor for LSPs if they were to address social exclusion, help regenerate neighbourhoods and reduce the 'health divide' for their local area. VCS members of health and wellbeing subgroups of the LSP commented on ways of improving public involvement in decision making and the VCS role in influencing priorities through the LSP. However, VCS members of health and wellbeing partnerships of the LSP emphasised the difficulties they faced in influencing partnerships. Not bringing money to partnerships meant that the VCS could be considered as an 'inferior partner'; decision making was described as taking place in the main LSP, rather than in its subgroups; and while the VCS was involved in delivering services, there was less influence on setting targets and agreeing priorities, especially in two-tier authorities. Finally engagement was often tokenistic and involvement of the public across all levels of decision making was difficult to achieve:

> 'It's more that the summit allows for the voluntary sector to be informed about what's happening in the partnership, but I think if I'm honest it's not exactly a two-way street at the moment so the influence of the sector, I think, is quite limited within the partnership.' (VCS member, site 8)

In two sites, VCS interviewees described themselves as playing a role in choosing local priorities and, in one of these, a third sector assembly had been established around themes of local area agreements (LAAs). VCS interviewees considered that a potential synergy between partnership strategies and the work of the VCS was not adequately exploited as partnerships were often unaware of activities carried out in the sector. This could lead to duplication, while opportunities to build on existing plans could be missed and commissioning decisions were not informed by intelligence from the VCS.

> 'I think most of the time they (VCS) spend just reacting and doing rather than thinking proactively about how they could get involved more in the strategic areas and how they fit with certain policies and strategic direction....They don't see how they fit with some of the targets, they don't see that they fit with the local area agreement and that some of the work that they're doing contributes to that.' (VCS member, site 4)

Interviewees described ways of improving partnership working at a local level although much depended on the local context. Locality networks of various kinds could span health and social care and the wider health agenda, and community assemblies could provide a focus for community views. Practice-based commissioners could also become involved on a locality basis. However, links across formal partnerships, such as the LSP and OSCs, were often poorly developed.

Public involvement in health scrutiny

In common with LSP subgroups, scrutiny committees were themed and each had a discrete remit, making it difficult to make links across different aspects of a health and wellbeing agenda. There were a few examples of scrutiny of health and wellbeing strategies, health inequalities and the LAAs, but, in general, there was little scrutiny of partnerships, of LAAs, of preventive services or of health protection. Instead the focus was largely on scrutiny of the health care system and of PCT targets and priorities, often in response to public concern. OSCs did not figure prominently in PCT accounts of governance and some interviewees argued that they did not present enough of a challenge to PCTs.

OSC interviewees concurred with VCS interviewees that public involvement in PCT decision making required development. However, Chairs of health scrutiny committees also described public involvement in the scrutiny function as minimal. One interviewee commented:

> 'Pretty poor, I'd say, because basically I would say most of the public would be completely unaware of the work of the scrutiny side of things. I think in my time I've chaired health for a year and a half, and we've had one deputation, which bearing in mind that would be the only way of the public getting involved, is pretty low.' (OSC chair, site 1)

Sites differed in the extent to which members of scrutiny committees sought out views of the public and in two sites there was a more proactive approach to public engagement. One interviewee described how they were improving engagement:

> 'So it's taking scrutiny into the community where it should be, not just tied up as we're sitting up in ivory towers so to speak and sending loads of literature out to people, a waste of time. You meet people face to face. ...' (OSC chair, site 6)

As part of this, it was argued the public needed to be more aware of how they could influence decision making. On the other hand, commissioners needed a better understanding of levers to promote communication and engagement with the populations that they served. A number of different routes were discussed including Mosaic profiling, working through umbrella VCS organisations or LINks, social marketing initiatives and raising the profile of the PCT. Other examples included face-to-face canvassing to increase public awareness of the health agenda and marketing routes through which the public could potentially influence commissioning decisions. There was therefore little evidence of a public health focus from OSCs, despite the expectations associated with them.

Relevance of the study to developments in public involvement

As mentioned earlier, LINks were abolished in 2013 and local Healthwatch took their place as the organisation designed to reflect the public voice in relation to local health and social care services. Although LINks was also an independent, statutory organisation, local Healthwatch is a core statutory member of the HWB (itself now a statutory subcommittee of the local authority) and is potentially in a stronger position to exert an influence on commissioners. Local Healthwatch representatives will be involved in developing JSNAs, for example, which was not the case for LINks in the study (with the exception of one site). However, concerns have been raised over certain elements of Healthwatch, including the lack of ring-fenced funding provided to councils, who are responsible for funding them, Healthwatch England's perceived lack of independence, due to its relationship with the CQC, and its capacity to support local Healthwatch.

Although local Healthwatch has to be a 'body corporate', there has been less prescription, which has led to a myriad of different organisational and legal forms (partly due to the complexity of local government procurement regulations). The relationship with local authorities has also changed significantly. As Healthwatch were designed to create a 'market' and to broaden the base of PPI, local authorities were able to put the local Healthwatch contracts out to tender with very clear specifications. It is likely that Healthwatch will be closely monitored by those who commissioned them, raising questions about their independence and ability to influence. There is little clarity as to their role and remit, particularly with respect to other monitoring bodies and lay representatives. Further, local Healthwatch is expected to work and network with the VCS (and the majority of local Healthwatch have been formed through collaborative partnerships within the voluntary sector). However, this may also lead to a focus on the group represented or a 'single issue' focus rather than action across the wider remit envisaged for local Healthwatch. As reflected in the study, the domination of 'single issues' and 'monopolisation' of the agenda by certain sectors of the VCS is likely to remain an issue, again rendering it hard to reflect the diversity of views.

There is also the added complexity of forging relationships with the former members of LINks who may not be represented in the new organisations. It may be difficult for local Healthwatch to find their 'niche' among the numerous mechanisms for engagement already established through local authorities. There are also inherent tensions in the organisational make-up of local Healthwatch. Concerns over the 'professionalising' of the third sector expressed in the study may be further exacerbated by the fact that many boards have been recruited externally, advertising for specific professional skills, thus potentially underlining the gap between the rhetoric and reality of engagement and, ironically, narrowing both its base and the possibility to reach wider audiences. In addition, similar to the development of LINks, simply transferring over to a new organisation may obscure a full understanding of the concept and remit of the new organisations and also, as a result, Healthwatch may not be able to fulfil its intended role or indeed the local authority specifications. On the other hand, there may be a danger of losing the LINks' 'capital' if there is not a transfer of people, information and skills.

Given this context, the development of local Healthwatch may signify a departure from the nature of PPI organisations that has developed over the last forty years but, importantly, such professionalisation and formalisation of PPI may be at the expense of both public and democratic accountability.

Conclusions

The complexities involved in achieving public involvement in health are well documented, as is the relative lack of success in achieving changes in services or organisations (Coleman et al., 2011). Whether related to health care service provision or wider decision making, public involvement in the NHS has often been described as tokenistic, with consultation sometimes taking place after decisions have been taken, where the capacity to change outcomes may have been limited from the outset, or where community views have been subsequently overturned or overruled. Research which has attempted to identify the impact of public involvement on management decisions has found limited impact (Harrison et al., 2002) and there was little engagement in commissioning despite the level of policy commitment. Coleman et al (2009: 28) comment that 'there is no clear agreement about what it means or how it can be achieved', arguing for a more contextual and contingent approach to addressing the complexities involved in public engagement. In an earlier study of the capacity of statutory organisations to work effectively with communities at a strategic level Pickin et al. (2002) emphasised the importance of transformational rather than transactional leadership styles and there is a tendency to underestimate the capacity building required for active citizenship (Jochum et al., 2005). As discussed in Chapter Two, participation is key for accountability and for 'good governance', yet locally there is a mix of governance arrangements which can lead to consultation overlap, confused accountability and lack of clarity over representation. Indeed, one of the reasons put forward for abolishing PPIFs and replacing them with LINks was their lack of diversity, with the majority of members being older adults and too few in number to represent the range of community views (House of Commons Health Committee, 2007).

The study showed variation in the ways in which LINks were established, a lack of clarity about their role and purpose, especially among GPs, some ambiguity in governance arrangements and problems of achieving representativeness. Issues of maintaining visibility and ensuring adequate feedback to members and wider community networks were key issues, as other studies have demonstrated (Melvin, 2010). These remain risks for the new organisations, although the lack of diversity in the make-up of local Healthwatch may be of a different nature. Nonetheless, the growing professionalisation of the third sector and specifically PPI organisations may enable a greater influence on the statutory sector. This would have implications for wider engagement and issues of representativeness and accountability.

As well as the question of how representative LINks had managed to become, their relationship with OSCs raised potential tensions between democratic decision making as reflected through local authorities and the complex issues of representativeness which arise in non-democratically elected organisations, of which LINks are an example. These tensions again remain with Healthwatch, required to raise concerns over local services with providers, commissioners and council health scrutiny committees. In the study, there was relatively little involvement of OSCs in scrutinising partnerships or preventive services. However, the potential complementarity of roles has been emphasised (Murphy and Turner, 2012: 11), with health scrutiny acting as a 'bridge between politicians, professionals and communities, so that solutions are identified together'.

From a governance perspective, a number of themes emerge from this chapter. First is a lack of clarity over the degree of influence to be exerted by PPI organisations in statutory organisations, as reflected in the varied involvement of LINks in PCT boards and subcommittees in the study. These themes are likely to persist as Healthwatch takes shape in the context of new commissioning arrangements. While CCGs are required to involve a lay member with experience of the local community, it is not clear how this relates to other decision-making structures across a local authority area or how much influence they will exert on CCG decision making. The Health and Social Care Bill 2012 mandates that a member of the local Healthwatch sits on the HWB, but there will be questions over how best to reflect local networks of voluntary organisations and negotiate the different types of accountability represented in these boards. Moreover, multi-district HWBs are likely to create added problems for local involvement. There are also questions of how much influence local Healthwatch will exert across different aspects of the commissioning cycle and whether they will also promote a preventive agenda or whether the focus will remain on local health and social care services.

Second, there are differences in how public involvement is being interpreted. It was clear from interviewees in four of the case study sites that while the PCTs were trying to involve the public in commissioning for health and wellbeing, there was little evidence of the public actually influencing commissioning decisions. PCT interviewees saw public involvement in commissioning as reflected through informal engagement activities with the public, while VCS interviewees expected more influence and direct formal involvement in decision making, a view expressed by one interviewee as follows:

> 'But when you ask public to be involved, engaged, their hopes are high, and they think they're going to alter or are able to alter the decision, whereas for the commissioners engagement means something else.' (VCS member, site 5)

This is likely to continue with the development of local Healthwatch, where their role in decision making and the commissioning process may be confined to their presence on HWBs, particularly in those areas where LINks personnel have not been transferred or where previous representation in commissioning was limited. It is equally notable that there also appears to be greater emphasis for Healthwatch to work with local networks, develop engagement processes, including community representatives, and collect views from the public rather than on being involved in commissioning. Coleman et al. (2011: 35) suggest there is a danger that as Healthwatch develops and deals with their new responsibilities, patient and public involvement is 'equated with providing information and allowing choice and the opportunity to embed meaningful democratic accountability is lost'.

Third, is the extent to which recurring questions of resources, membership and remit raised by the House of Commons Health Committee (2007) in relation to LINks will be resolved in local Healthwatch. Finally and paradoxically, increased public involvement in decision making may not necessarily result in a greater emphasis on public health and preventive services. The provision of health and social care services commands a higher public profile and is of more immediate concern to the public. This may, however, be counterbalanced by a greater emphasis on asset-based approaches in local communities, and the relocation of public health commissioning in democratically elected local authorities.

The study demonstrated that more effective and systematic involvement in commissioning was needed and illustrated a number of barriers to achieving this, especially in relation to a preventive agenda. When public spending is being reduced and difficult decisions are being made over disinvestment, it will be even more important to demonstrate transparency and to develop more effective ways of involving the public in commissioning processes, including those for priority setting.

CHAPTER EIGHT

Conclusions

Through mutual concerns with social justice, the human right to health and the health of populations, 'good governance' can be seen as inextricably linked to a public health agenda. Understanding governance in relation to public health is therefore inseparable from wider debates over governance, the extent to which underlying governance principles are reflected in practice and implications of the balance adopted across different kinds of governance arrangements. Relationships between governance and health can be considered for each of the different dimensions of governance – principles of governance, various governance arrangements and modes of governance – so that, for example, questions can be raised over the extent to which the principle of social justice is reflected in national policy, in local public health initiatives and monitored through health equity audit, or the extent to which the principle of accountability is reflected in levels of public involvement and engagement.

Relationships between governance and health can also be considered across national, regional and local levels of decision making, or in relation to global governance. Drawing on empirical research, this book illustrates the relevance of dimensions of governance for commissioning for health and wellbeing at a local level.

Much attention has been directed to 'steering' instruments, such as performance management regimes or the use of incentives, and their effectiveness in improving outcomes in public services. Questions include the balance to be achieved across regulatory approaches and devolved decision making, the effectiveness of incentives and the costs and benefits of different approaches to performance management. At the time of the study, steering instruments included national guidance, policy priorities, public service agreements (PSAs) and other national and local targets, all of which were reflected in the assessment activities of regulatory agencies. The study focused on the influence of such arrangements on commissioning for health and wellbeing and showed that the complex system of targets and governance arrangements which framed decision making within commissioning organisations did not meet the aims of government policies for prevention. Even where relevant policies and targets were in place, such as for addressing health inequalities, this proved little guarantee of implementation, as there were contextual influences, competing priorities, and not all targets were subjected to the same level of scrutiny. Performance management arrangements were widely viewed as ill aligned, focused on specific organisations rather than on the partnerships required to promote health across a local area, and weighted towards national rather than local targets. However, this should not be taken to imply that performance management arrangements should be abandoned. Policy commitments for improving population health or addressing health inequalities are unlikely to prove successful unless they are reflected throughout governance arrangements and decision-making processes at national, regional and local levels. They were seen by some interviewees as a spur to local performance and arguably, without a degree of measurement, scrutiny or performance management in relation to public health, there would be little scope to gauge how far governments were reflecting 'good governance' in relation to the stewardship of population health.

Nevertheless, at the time of the study, the emphasis on targets and delivery chains to deliver public service outcomes led to tensions between devolved priority setting on the one hand and centralised monitoring to encourage improved performance on the other. The importance of local-level governance was emphasised through focus groups in the study and linked to an ability to develop creative and locally relevant modes of delivery, and to shift from a predominant focus on organisational governance to a 'governance of place'. Where local targets had been developed, these could act as a powerful lever for change:

> 'No one really cares how we do in relation to someone else, but in the city, the councillors, everyone else, are thinking about their relevance to local people, you do care about that and also you live there and that affects ... how you think of your city as a place. That drive to localism is a really powerful governance lever.' (National focus group in Marks et al., 2010: 58)

Devolving decision making to a local level has been emphasised by the coalition government and is reflected in a less centralised system of performance management. However, previous health-related targets through PSAs had largely been met (or progress made), with the exceptions of deterioration in the health inequalities target (despite increases in life expectancy in absolute terms), patient experience, and limited progress on under-18 teenage conception rates (King's Fund, n.d.). The impact on health outcomes of the decision by the coalition government to abandon many of the targets and performance management arrangements put in place by the preceding Labour government has yet to be assessed.

As for incentive arrangements in relation to preventive services, there was recognition in the study of the dangers of piecemeal and uncoordinated approaches. Incentives included in baseline budgets were ineffective and rewards for reducing demand could hardly be considered as incentives if they were contingent on the overall financial situation of the commissioning organisation. Transactional approaches to change could be effective in the short term, but their impact was limited and the quality of leadership, organisational support for achieving change and a sense of commitment also acted as important incentives, as did the governance arrangements in place. The potential for incentives to have perverse and unintended consequences, either directly or indirectly (through conflicting incentives across a system), were recognised: debates over incentives intended to promote public health continue in the context of the intention, at the time of writing, to offer a 'Health Premium' for local authority performance for improving local outcomes. Payment by results continues to act as an incentive for increasing activity in the acute sector.

In addition to the traditional triumvirate of markets, networks and hierarchies, modes of governance such as co-governance, partnership governance and participatory governance are particularly important for addressing system-wide changes needed to address complex public health challenges. Gostin and Stone (2007) argue, for example, for a new public health ethic, committed to 'ideas of community and partnership'. Modes of governance raise questions related to their potential impact on health outcomes, in particular the effect of competition (through markets) and its effects on coordination and integrated working. Market modes of governance have been associated with increasing health inequalities and with reductions in equitable access to services, while the relative emphasis on hierarchical or networked modes of governance may affect the development of local partnerships or cross-sectoral working. In the study, a market mode of governance was also considered to work against the involvement of the smaller voluntary organisations, for example, which would find it difficult to compete, despite their level of engagement with underserved groups.

The importance of partnerships and of participatory governance is reflected in the arrangements, from April 2013, for statutory health and wellbeing boards (HWBs), which bring together local authorities, clinical commissioning groups (CCGs) and local community organisations. Much is expected from these new boards, which will face well-documented challenges involved in agreeing priorities and coordinating action across agencies with different budgets and accountability arrangements. Challenges related to both partnership governance and participatory governance were illustrated in the study. It showed, for example, that performance management arrangements encouraged success within, rather than across organisations and that engagement of partners in public health-related activities was variable. While CCGs are core members of HWBs, involvement of general practice in the commissioning process and in public health partnerships was minimal at the time of the study (although there were some exceptions). This was particularly the case in developing joint strategic needs assessments (JSNAs), now a key focus for HWBs. For practice-based commissioners, the focus remained on business plans, demand management and care pathway redesign. Moreover, practice-based commissioning (PBC) largely relied on a small number of enthusiasts, the provider role remained dominant and there were concerns over how easy it would be for conflicts of interest across provider and commissioner roles to be resolved. There is, therefore, a risk that demand management and a focus on the integration of health and social care may narrow the focus of HWBs, and that conflicts of interest over the commissioner and provider role may re-emerge.

Participatory governance is clearly placed on a stronger footing through the democratic legitimacy of local councils and their engagement with local populations, but the study reflected difficulties involved in ensuring representativeness of the voluntary and community sector (VCS) or in demonstrating actual influence on commissioning decisions. While public involvement was encouraged through world class commissioning (WCC), public engagement in a public health agenda was often difficult to achieve and influence on commissioning decisions was considered to be minimal. There were also difficulties in achieving a balance across local responsiveness and the economies of scale required for effective commissioning.

While the impact of each mode of governance can be considered separately, there are wider debates over the mix of different modes of governance which obtain at a particular time and to what extent they encourage the achievement of policy goals. For many public health problems, relationships between cause and effect are complex and may not be completely understood. Addressing them involves action on the part of different sectors and agencies – across a whole system. This raises questions over approaches to governance best suited to complex systems, characterised by unpredictability and dispersed responsibilities.

Equally important as considering different dimensions of governance is the extent to which there is coherence across them. Principles of governance are intended to inform governance arrangements, and a failure to achieve 'governance coherence' can undermine the best policy intentions and contribute to an implementation gap between policy and practice. The study showed that commissioners make decisions in the context of complex and sometimes conflicting incentives and governance arrangements. National targets for prevention were not always prioritised in practice and resources earmarked for prevention could easily be re-routed as other priorities emerged. Public health investment was often contingent on other priorities and targets having been met, on growth money being available, with prevention often described as an 'earned agenda'. At a local level, the WCC cycle was designed to encourage a coherent approach to commissioning, backed up by an assurance process and this, to some extent at least, was reflected in corporate governance arrangements. However, unforeseen problems (typically resource constraints) worked against the implementation of local strategic plans. A fundamental problem was that of conflicting incentives within the health system, in particular the paradox of encouraging increases in acute sector activity through the system of payment by results while at the same time encouraging demand management in primary care, which was intended to achieve the opposite.

Taking a 'whole system' approach enables a better appreciation of the interplay of incentives in different parts of the system and of the extent to which governance arrangements and the particular combination of modes of governance (such as markets and partnerships) may reflect conflicting goals. The importance of considering governance as a whole has been demonstrated through scandals arising from governance failures. In Mid Staffordshire NHS Foundation Trust, for example (Francis Inquiry, 2013), an emphasis on one area of governance (in this case achieving financial targets required for achieving Foundation Trust status) deflected attention from the broader principles and purpose of the organisation. One of the recommendations of the final report in 2013 was a more coherent approach to governance arrangements:

> There should be a single regulator dealing both with corporate governance, financial competence, viability and compliance with patient safety and quality standards for all trusts', thereby recognising a fragmentation of regulation which prevented a coherent overview of governance arrangements. (Recommendation 19)

Leadership involves the ability to understand and negotiate complex governance arrangements and their relationship to the purpose of the organisation. Leadership for population health is inevitably complex as it involves working with different organisations and in partnership with multiple stakeholders at different levels, engaging with local communities and understanding the different types of accountability in place. In the study, it was emphasised that governance in relation to population health was not located within a single partnership or governance arrangement but involved leadership for incorporating a public health perspective across other departments with their own governance arrangements:

> 'And in many senses I think the challenge for local champions of health improvement is to try and build health dimensions into all of the governance structures – for children's trusts, for programmes around social care, for crime and disorder partnerships, for all of the other activities that you've got, which have got fairly well firmed up governance structures of their own.' (National focus group)

The study showed the importance of committed leadership if performance management arrangements were not to be the subject of gaming or otherwise subverted. The dispersed model of public health leadership across the local authority and the primary care trust (PCT) at the time of the study was perceived as counterproductive by some interviewees.

At a local level, while there was an emphasis in WCC on future orientation and on investing for health over the longer term, in practice, shorter-term health care priorities predominated. In addition, PCTs and local authorities had different perspectives over the relative emphasis that should be accorded to behavioural interventions or social determinants of health. One interviewee described the contrast as follows:

> 'Someone who really focuses on world class commissioning, PCT agenda and kind of really focused on perhaps the integration of all the healthy lifestyle work, sort of behavioural, a bit of weight management, all that kind of stuff. And then you have someone in the local authority who actually is the one who kind of talks about the health impacts of what is going on in the local authority, and about shaping the environment and regeneration and local

development frameworks and spatial policies and all those sorts of things. I don't think you can satisfactorily do the two things.' (Deputy director of public health [DPH], site 5)

Where principles of governance, such as social equity, are not adopted or are inadequately reflected in governance arrangements, public health leadership may require an advocacy role, as well as 'due diligence' in relation to emerging problems and an 'anticipatory' approach to governance (Fuerth, 2009). It has been argued, for example (Graham, 2010), that the public health system lacks anticipation of future conditions, their potential impact on health and on intergenerational inequalities, and that the concentration on immediate risks and short-term benefits takes its cue from short-term political objectives. She argues that this perspective is reflected in approaches to evidence, where evidence from randomised controlled trials is ill suited not only to identifying the impact of complex interventions but also for assessing the impact of environmental changes which affect whole populations. These themes were reflected in the study, where focus group participants argued that programme management had overshadowed policy analysis and the health consequences of policy decisions: value-led interventions were also important:

> 'Now all of those things [libraries, parks and schools] have been created in places where there was no evidence base, no sort of randomised controlled trial. They've been created on the basis of critical values and all of those, and a wide range of other things have a profound impact on people's health. So I think the notion of value-led interventions is equally important.' (National focus group)

A study of the capacity of managers to manage for health (Marks and Hunter, 2005) suggested that 'public health governance' could be used as a short-hand term for the critical assessment of the range of governance approaches as they related to public health (singly and in combination). However, as illustrated in Chapter One, both governance and public health are open to multiple interpretations. 'Public health' can refer to population health, a public health system (which may be broadly or narrowly defined), a public health workforce or the main types of activity carried out by public health practitioners, and the interpretation of public health governance can vary accordingly. In the same way, 'governance' can be used to refer to various 'steering instruments' or can encompass the broader principles of 'good governance', including social justice. For example, the phrase 'public health governance' has been used to refer to regulatory approaches to public health as well as to governance arrangements related to core activities and standards of public health practitioners. In the study, public health governance was sometimes identified with complying with the existing governance arrangements of an organisation. To combine 'public health' with 'governance' therefore risks multiplying ambiguity. A holistic approach to public health governance could encompass the impact of all the dimensions of governance, as described Chapter Two, and identify governance arrangements and approaches most suited to particular public health issues. This would inevitably involve ethical debates, including those over the balance across regulatory and other approaches to improving health. This perspective provides a much needed focus on public health, and also allows for the identification of 'governance deficits' (as well as governance successes), drawing on the extent of avoidable morbidity and mortality, health inequalities or the capacity to anticipate public health problems.

Governance deficits in public health

Just as failures in corporate governance informed a better understanding of what was required for 'good governance' in organisations, and poor quality clinical care acted as a trigger for developing clinical governance, failures in public health can inform the parameters of public health governance. As well as being reflected in levels of preventable morbidity and premature mortality, this deficit can manifest itself in an imbalance between 'upstream' and 'downstream' interventions; a failure to prioritise the prevention of ill health (or to adequately reflect this in resource allocation); the persistence and worsening of health inequalities; lack of anticipatory governance or of modelling future health risks; and in varying levels of partnership and of citizen engagement.

There is clearly no room for complacency. Despite wide-ranging policies, targets and standards devoted to commissioning for improved health outcomes, the Global Burden of Disease study (Murray et al., 2013) demonstrated that the performance of the UK (between 1990 and 2010) in terms of premature mortality was 'persistently and significantly' below the mean of 15 countries (where the original members of the European Union were chosen for comparison), despite an increase in life expectancy as measured in absolute terms. The authors considered 'additional action' was required to counter preventable morbidity and mortality, including leadership to ensure a 'multisectoral integrated response'. The emphasis on the multisectoral response reiterates the importance of locating public health governance within a wider system, if factors influencing health and health equity are to be addressed.

The Wanless reports (2002, 2004) drew attention to the importance of citizen engagement as part of a third and 'fully engaged' scenario, which would promote population health and reduce health care costs. Despite a nearly 50% increase in NHS funding being premised on this third scenario and implemented by the Labour government, projected savings from improved population health did not materialise. An update (Wanless et al., 2007) showed that certain measures of morbidity, such as long-standing illness, remained unchanged and that inequalities had increased. The report also pointed out that it was not possible to track trends in health promotion spending given a lack of data, or to identify whether the aspiration of a doubling of expenditure on public health had been met. Evidence from qualitative research corroborated the view that public health budgets, including resources earmarked for public health activities in the White Paper, *Choosing health* (Secretary of State for Health, 2004), were seen as easy pickings and frequently raided in order to order to meet other targets or to ease financial deficits (Hunter et al., 2010). The persistence of the inequalities gap has since been detailed for England (Marmot Review, 2010), Europe (Marmot et al., 2012) and globally (WHO, 2008).

If stewardship of population health, health equity and participation are considered hallmarks of good governance, then governance deficits in public health are also indicators of wider failures of governance. These issues were discussed in the focus groups carried out as part of the study where participants highlighted the lack of appropriate and timely action in relation to emerging public health hazards; a failure to identify public health consequences of public policy decisions (either singly or in combination); and a narrow approach to effectiveness, bolstered by a limited conception of what constitutes an evidence base in public health. However, this raises questions over the primacy of health and health equity in decisions taken in other sectors which may have a bearing on health and the extent to which health (and health inequalities) impact assessments are carried out and then acted on.

Moral and ethical issues which arise from societal approaches to protecting and promoting health at a group or population level are reflected in the field of public health ethics (Kass, 2004; Dawson and Verweij, 2007; Gostin, 2008; Peckham and Hann, 2009). As discussed in the introduction, stewardship can refer to the collective responsibility governments assume for protecting the health of the population (Saltman and Ferroussier-Davis, 2000; WHO, 2000) and it has been suggested that improving healthy life expectancy should be an overarching policy goal against which other policies are judged (Bernstein et al., 2010). However, the parameters of a stewardship role are framed by ethical and political debates over the balance to be negotiated across individual and collective responsibility (Jochelson, 2005), across public and private interests, or the rights of the community over individual freedoms. Kass (2001) identifies two facets: 'a code of restraint', to ensure the rights of citizens in relation to the powers of the state, and 'affirmative obligations to improve the public's health'. Ethical issues which arise include the extent of personal responsibility for health (which may be reflected in the policy balance across regulation and persuasion), how priorities are reached within existing resources, the balance negotiated between maximising and equalising population health and targeting high-risk groups versus universal population-based approaches (Brock, 2007; Wikler and Brock, 2007). In its discussion of the implications of a stewardship model (and reflecting the association of stewardship with equity and social justice) the Nuffield Council on Bioethics (2007: v) characterised a 'stewardship-guided state' as holding a 'particular responsibility for protecting the health of vulnerable groups such as children, and in closing the gap between the most and least healthy in society'. It highlighted the role of corporate social responsibility in public health and argued, for example, that the food industry has an ethical duty to help individuals make healthier food choices and that governments should step in with legislation if it fails to do so. For alcohol, the report suggests that the stewardship model would imply more coercive measures in areas of price, marketing and availability than those which currently hold sway. It suggested an ethical framework for a 'stewardship-guided state', developing an eight-rung 'intervention ladder' for considering the justification for different public health policies and instruments (ranging from eliminating choice to simple monitoring). The more coercive the measure, the stronger the justification needed.

It has been argued that public health ethics can act as a 'call to arms' for a reinvigorated approach to decision making for collective wellbeing. Global justice, environmental ethics and greater commitment to public health research have all been included under its rubric (Kass, 2004) and, more recently, government responses to austerity that are hazardous to population health and increase inequalities have been reframed as questions of ethics as well as of economics (Stuckler and Basu, 2013).

Local commissioning for health and wellbeing post-2013

The implementation of the Health and Social Care Act 2012 meant a major shift in accountability for public health, with local authorities responsible for improving the health of their populations and held accountable through local elections, to their populations. Public health teams (and a ring-fenced public health grant) were transferred from the NHS to local authorities This meant that the NHS was no longer accountable for the delivery of a wide range of local public health services.

HWBs were established on a statutory basis as a committee of the local authority and charged with taking a strategic overview across partners in the light of the findings of the JSNA. The engagement of GPs in commissioning was formalised through the development of CCGs and the former indicative budgets of practice-based commissioners were replaced with legal budgetary responsibility. New accountability arrangements were established through NHS England (at national and regional levels), Public Health England and CCG governing bodies. Despite the intentions of creating a less centralised and complex system, Maybin et al. (2011) point to the potential for hierarchical control of CCGs by NHS England, while the weak internal governance mechanisms for HWBs and CCGs are likely to lead to accountability problems. They note the 'shift to an over-reliance on weak and unproven accountability relationships' (p. ix).

The relocation of responsibility of public health to local authorities has been largely welcomed as recognising the influence on health and health inequalities of social determinants of health, the importance of decision making within a framework of democratic accountability and the capacity to engage with local communities. This was also reflected in the study where a focus group participant noted that:

> 'I personally believe that the notion of joint DsPH, while it is sort of held up as the answer is just a way station to DsPH ending up completely back inside local government. I think they are still on a journey and the more they embed themselves, the more they'll realise that actually the place to be is in local government and not in the NHS.'

The shift into local authorities and therefore into a system of democratic accountability means a change in decision-making contexts and processes, including the development of different criteria for priority setting. It is likely to promote a focus on upstream interventions aligned to the public health influence of other local authority directorates rather than on secondary prevention and the predominantly lifestyle-based approach of PCTs. Focus groups in the study argued for a different balance between social and clinical interventions, for example, enabling people with mental health problems to find work, or ensuring that the link between debt and mental health was reflected in integrated packages of primary care which included debt counselling advice:

> 'The evidence base around bigger income equals better health is much stronger than many of the other things the commissioners buy. So it would be that kind of interrogation really of the system.' (National focus group)

Case studies from the experience of the first nine months of the reforms, jointly commissioned by the Local Government Association and Public Health England, illustrated innovative ways in which councils were developing their public health role (Local Government Association, 2014). In a foreword, Sir Merrick Cockell, chair of the Local Government Association, noted that local authorities were developing:

> a new culture in which health is at the heart of integrated planning and services, in which all parts of the council and all of the providers delivering services on the council's behalf understand how they can contribute to better public health outcomes. (Local Government Association, 2014: 3)

There were examples of 'whole council' approaches to public health; health impact assessments of local policies; developing integrated health and wellbeing services; involving other council directorates in delivering the public health outcomes framework; and DsPH taking on wider roles in the council. At the same time, differences in culture and organisation were recognised, with greater weight being attached within local authorities to the priorities of local citizens. While the reforms may have acted as a catalyst for change in local authorities and a greater leadership role in public health it is also the case that local authorities have always played a key role in improving health and influencing local determinants of health through their responsibilities for housing, the environment, transport and education. Many could also build on a long history of joint working with PCTs and of jointly appointed DsPH.

For the time being, there is less focus on national targets and performance management, and more encouragement of local decision making and self-assessment, through outcomes frameworks for public health, social care and health care. These changes also imply greater variation, as changes in the political composition of local authorities are likely to influence approaches adopted to narrow health inequalities and less central control through performance management may also lead to greater local variation.

The focus on a commissioning cycle, as promoted through WCC, has changed although the emphasis on JSNAs, as the starting point of that cycle, has been maintained and arguably strengthened through the statutory role of the HWB in developing JSNAs and coordinating implementation through joint health and wellbeing strategies. It is not clear to what extent the lack of interest in JSNAs shown in the study on the part of GP practices will persist. Dangers of the JSNA degenerating into a purely technical exercise were highlighted in focus groups in the study:

> 'But it's also ensuring that within the strategic needs assessment, it's not just simply facts, it actually contains an analysis of what the local drivers are, what the local motivators are, what the local influencing processes are, because that's actually the bit that helps you to translate hard information into something that actually becomes useful, and can be used by people.' (National focus group)

There is potential for the JSNA to become more central in commissioning decisions and, in particular, for the public to become more engaged in developing the JSNA, which could better reflect community assets as well as community 'deficits' (Foot and Hopkins, 2010).

While different stages of a commissioning cycle are generic, the context for decision making has changed. For PCTs, which held commissioning responsibilities across health care and preventive services, there was potential flexibility for shifting the 'gravity of spend' towards prevention across a care pathway or across total spend, with the incentive of reducing health care costs if effective preventive initiatives were implemented. Lifestyle interventions, clinical preventive services and secondary prevention were prioritised in PCTs over primary prevention, mainly because of the evidence base for their impact on health over the shorter term and their relationship to the core business of the health service, but possibly also by a potential payback from reduced demand for health care services. They were also able to support GP practices in developing preventive services. This focus has changed as public health is more clearly located in social conditions, local decision making and planning decisions across different local authority responsibilities. Local authorities are well placed to get best value for prevention out of local authority spend, but incentives for prioritising preventive services may be lessened. At the same time, the role of CCGs in behavioural interventions may become more limited. While arguments for demonstrating a return on investment are likely to continue, there will be potential for increased emphasis on identifying the health impact of policies across local authority directorates and a greater focus on local accountability for the decisions made. In the study, there were many examples of innovative commissioning practice but there is a danger that much of the experience of commissioning preventive services will be lost with the demise of PCTs. Maintaining public health networks and developing more effective methods for knowledge exchange will be equally important under the new arrangements.

While the study illustrated the difficulties of partnership working across the local authority and PCTs, achieving joined-up governance for localities through the members of HWBs is likely to remain challenging. The study showed that there was a tendency to define health and wellbeing as the sum total of NHS activities. This argument can equally be applied by local authorities, in that the gamut of council services can also be argued to enhance health and wellbeing. The danger remains of a longer-term preventive agenda being lost as immediate priorities predominate. Leadership for public health and the ability to tell a 'compelling story' will be important. In the context of local authorities this leadership will reside in elected councillors as members of the council Cabinet and be reflected in Cabinet decision making.

At a local level, much will depend on how health and wellbeing are understood, how the contribution to health across different agencies is recognised and aligned, and the extent to which a public health agenda is prioritised and then implemented by those who decide how resources are to be spent. However, room for manoeuvre will inevitably be limited by the cuts in public spending, with preventive services often the first to suffer during periods of economic decline. The impact of the credit crunch on NHS finances post 2010/11 was clear in the second phase of the study, with an emphasis on efficiency savings, prioritisation strategies for investment and, increasingly, disinvestment, and less opportunity to develop and evaluate innovative health promoting programmes. In practice, resources intended for public health have often been viewed as easy pickings, especially in times of financial stringency.

At national and international levels, population health and the prevention of avoidable ill health are inextricably linked with commitments to social justice and the development of health–informed public policy and, as such, to broader questions of governance and of stewardship. Local decision making with an impact on population health and health equity is also influenced by the depth of commitment to social justice and a preventive ethos. However, it does not exist in isolation from this national context which, in turn, influences priorities and governance arrangements. Using the governance framework described in this book may help to identify whether governance principles and the arrangements which reflect them are being brought together at national and local levels to achieve effective 'public health governance'.

Study methods and case study snapshots

The study *Public health governance and primary care delivery: A triangulated study* was carried out from 2007 to 2010 and funded by the National Institute for Health Research Service Delivery and Organisation public health research programme.[1] The study adopted mixed methods, drawing together quantitative and qualitative analysis from a range of research activities. An initial exploratory phase involved one national and two regional focus groups across England, and mapping and scoping exercises, including reviews of economic perspectives on incentives, prioritisation tools, public health governance and performance management arrangements in force at the time, including targets, standards and incentives. Fieldwork was carried out in 10 case study sites across England, selected to reflect different levels of disadvantage, urban and rural areas, a range of population size and different levels of performance in relation to public health targets.

A total of 99 interviews were carried out between 2008 and 2010, in two phases, one year apart. Participants included primary care trust (PCT) chief executives, chairs and other non-executive directors, directors of commissioning, finance and public health; practice-based commissioning (PBC) leads; professional executive committee (PEC) chairs; chairs of local overview and scrutiny committees (OSCs) for health; voluntary and community sector (VCS) representatives on health and wellbeing partnerships of the local strategic partnership and chairs of the recently formed local involvement networks (LINks). Documentary analysis was also carried out for each site. In order to locate case study findings in a national context, a national survey of PCTs was sent to 508 individuals across 146/152 PCTs (some shared boards) with responses from 65% of PCTs. The report drew together findings from qualitative and quantitative studies from the different phases of research, locating fieldwork in a national context and interpreting data in a governance framework. A brief summary of case study snapshots is included below to provide a context for study findings.

Case study sites

Site 1: an ethnically and culturally diverse PCT with a population of over 250,000. Life expectancy was higher than the English average but rates of TB and diabetes were high, as was child poverty and homelessness. There was a high population turnover. The director of public health (DPH) was a joint appointment with the local authority and public health was well integrated into governance arrangements and strategic development. Resources for prevention, including those for smoking cessation, had been cut back during a period of financial difficulty but were being reinstated. The majority of GPs were in single or two-handed practices, but primary care needed development and there was relatively limited use of incentives (through local enhanced services (LES)) for preventive services. As in other sites, investment in prevention was contingent on managing demand for acute services. Skills in using decision-making tools were considered in short supply. Making the business case for health and wellbeing remained difficult, given problems in quantifying long-term benefit, compounded by the fact of a highly mobile population. Patient and public involvement in the PCT needed development: there were cultural, educational and language barriers to public involvement, and social marketing was being developed to try to improve take up of preventive services. Local priorities were considered inadequately reflected in nationally driven performance management regimes.

Site 2: a rural PCT with a population of almost 700,000, spanning one county council and numerous districts. There were pockets of deprivation, but better health than the England average. The PCT had recently moved into financial balance. Each authority had a local strategic partnership (LSP), which created difficulties in agreeing priorities, negotiating across county and district targets and finding the resources to participate. There was proactive public health input into commissioning, including practice-based and locality-based commissioning. PBC, although variable, had developed innovative preventive services and a county-wide data repository had facilitated development of the joint strategic needs assessment (JSNA), which was considered well integrated into decision making. There were pooled budgets with the local authority for health and wellbeing, and a substantial health and wellbeing fund for deprived areas, managed through the local authority and funded by the PCT. PBC clusters had public health representatives and cluster-specific public health reports. There had been a year-long exercise to engage the public in principles and criteria for investment in the health and wellbeing agenda, using different consultation methods, including focus groups, but the LINk was poorly developed. The PCT was considered proactive in engaging with the VCS and innovative approaches for reaching young people were being developed.

Site 3: a PCT with a population of just under 230,000 and a younger profile than the national average. Health was similar to the England average but with significant inequalities within the PCT and relatively high smoking levels. The PCT was coterminous with the unitary authority. It had recently moved into financial stability but tight budget management was in place. Commissioning for health and wellbeing was described as core for the organisation: there was a public health-led approach to commissioning, reflected in strategic development, methods for defining and tracking preventative health spend, and a commitment to increase preventative health spend by a certain percentage each year. Extensive use had been made of programme budgeting. LESs were increasingly used for incentivising preventive services in primary care. Joint appointments across the PCT and the local authority were emphasised, although a period of instability in the local authority had served to undermine partnerships and joint commissioning. The JSNA had benefited from a shared data observatory, but there was little involvement of PBC. PBC was considered well developed but it had resulted in few changes to commissioning. The LINk was particularly active, including at PCT board level, where the chair was a non-voting member, and LINk members were involved in working groups, tender panels, specifications and pathway redesign. Involvement of the LINk with the local authority was less well developed and there were tensions across the LINk and an overarching VCS group. As in other sites, relationships across the LINk and the LSP were underdeveloped.

Site 4 covered two local authorities, with a population of almost 300,000. Health was worse than the England average with high smoking rates and extensive health inequalities: life expectancy was amongst the worst in the country for one of the boroughs. The DPH was jointly appointed across both boroughs. A sound financial footing had made it possible to make additional investments in health and wellbeing. There was a public health model of commissioning and addressing health inequalities was described as 'centre stage', with the PCT chair taking an active role in both of the health and wellbeing partnerships. Some considered targets essential to shift the focus towards health and wellbeing. There had been extensive public consultation for the JSNA but there were some problems over integration and sharing of health and local authority data. Alignment of PBC schemes with local priorities had been achieved through increased public health input into PBC consortia but they had not developed health and wellbeing initiatives. As in most other sites, links between PBC and JSNAs were not well developed. LINks were still being established, building on former patient and public involvement forums. As in other sites, the VCS was keen to have stronger voice in decision making.

Site 5: an inner-city PCT, coterminous with the local authority and with a population of just over 200,000. Health was below the England average with high levels of obesity and child poverty. The PCT had moved into financial stability. Leadership was consistently described as good or 'inspirational', with increased investment in partnership working and strategy development with the local authority and also with the VCS. This was reflected in a locality focus, bringing together service providers, residents and councillors. There had been a major shift towards improving health and tackling health inequalities, largely funded through growth money. Improving access and quality in primary care and better contract management were emphasised. The JSNA, developed with wide engagement, was described as an important catalyst for investment. As in other sites, there were differences in the ways that health needs assessment was understood across the local authority and the PCT, and debate about the extent to which the JSNA informed PBC priorities. The emphasis on collaboration across practices was reflected in plans to develop federated networks aligned with local partnerships. LESs were widely used to incentivise preventive care, but there was scepticism about achieving change through a contractual approach. Although slow to become established, the LINk had wide membership and was also represented on the PCT board. A large VCS was widely used to identify local health needs, contribute to strategy development and provide services, such as smoking cessation and health trainers. As in other sites, the focus was on prioritising growth money rather than across total spend and there was concern over the impact of financial stringency on the preventive agenda.

Site 6 was coterminous with a metropolitan borough, with a population of around 300,000. Health was worse than the average for England with marked health inequalities. Public health was described as embedded throughout the commissioning process, with strong public health leadership. Growth funds/financial surplus were identified for 'health turnaround', mainly for preventive services, and funds for health inequalities had been guaranteed for two years. Some preventive services delivered by the VCS had been jointly commissioned with the local Council for Voluntary Services and the VCS was widely used for providing health promotion services. The JSNA included community profiles, with enhanced profiles for disadvantaged areas, and had encouraged data sharing across the PCT and local authority. There was some joint commissioning with the local authority (for example, exercise on prescription and healthy school meals). The LINk was only recently established and there were no formal links with the LSP or with JSNA development. All practices were involved in PBC, and were provided with health profiles but there was little involvement in developing the JSNA. LESs were considered the most effective way of providing additional preventive services in primary care, although there were attempts to rationalise their use. Public involvement was encouraged through patient involvement on planning boards as well as through stakeholder events and community conferences where public health profiles of communities were shared. Members of the public were reimbursed for their involvement in PCT meetings. However, involvement in strategic decision making was relatively limited.

Site 7: an urban PCT with a population of over half a million and coterminous with a city council. Health was close to the English average although inequalities within the PCT persisted and a number of areas remained worse than average. PCT organisation reflected the commissioning cycle and the DPH, a joint appointment, had developed innovative approaches to targeting disadvantaged communities through enhanced public health programmes. However, as in other sites, shifting investment into public health was dependent on achieving financial balance, meeting national targets and then deploying efficiency savings from other parts of the health care system. A joint DPH and JSNA report had been developed (2008), but greater involvement of the VCS, the public and PBC was required along with stronger links between practices and multi-agency work in localities. It made commissioning recommendations for both the PCT and PBC. PBC was described as making good progress with the emphasis, as in other sites, on developing clinical pathways of care. There was no structure for involving the public in PBC. Despite some scepticism, LESs were considered an effective way of achieving results in general practice. Patient and public involvement was well developed, with examples of direct involvement in commissioning. The LINk had also made good progress, although its constituency was described as 'diffused'. While there were close links across LINks and the OSC, there were few with PBC, the LSP or with JSNA development. Programme budgeting data was used for benchmarking and health economics modelling was being carried out.

Site 8: an urban PCT with a population of over 350,000. It was not coterminous with the city council and partnerships with the local authority required further development. Health was worse than the English average. There was a city-wide health and wellbeing partnership but the DPH was not a joint appointment, although there were some joint roles. Public health was involved in commissioning health improvement services rather than being embedded throughout the commissioning cycle. Health and wellbeing was given a high priority in the PCT, with an emphasis on developing innovative approaches for self-management of long-term conditions. Engagement with local populations was being developed through social marketing initiatives, informed by geo-demographic tools, such as Mosaic. The JSNA was city wide and there had been extensive consultation, including a citizen's panel and some engagement with LINks and the VCS. However, there had been little involvement of PBC. A DPH report made commissioning recommendations and argued that locality commissioning boards were integral to commissioning for health and wellbeing. PBC localities developed three-year locality commissioning development plans. LESs were being reduced as they had often been used for funding mainstream services and were inadequately performance managed: developing innovative approaches through new contracts and partnerships was considered more fruitful. There were VCS networks and a third sector assembly, which had been involved in the choice of targets. Strategic involvement in the commissioning process by the VCS was described as needing development: VCS interviewees argued that the PCTs and partnerships needed greater awareness of knowledge held through the VCS. Setting up the LINk had been a slow process and representativeness had been difficult to achieve.

Site 9: a population of just over 300,000 and better health than the English average, although there were marked health inequalities. It was not coterminous with the local authority. The PCT was financially stable and health and wellbeing had been funded primarily through growth money. The DPH was a joint appointment. Public health and addressing health inequalities were described as central to the PCT, reflected throughout the commissioning process, and organisational structures were shifting to reflect commissioning functions. The JSNA, largely council led, had involved a large consultation exercise and the public was also involved in a strategic commissioning forum and in priority setting. The DPH report made commissioning recommendations but neither the JSNA nor the DPH report considered PBC, nor how the JSNA would influence local authority commissioning. Progress in PBC was consistently described as good: pooling arrangements were in place across clusters to allow resources to be used for larger schemes and, unusually, freed-up resources were made recurrent. LESs were seen as a successful way of incentivising changes in primary care, although it was argued that more effective use of contractual levers was needed. The PCT had also used individual incentives to motivate changes in behaviour. Public involvement was encouraged through a public consultation event before each PCT board meeting. The LSP held an annual stakeholder event for the VCS, which was involved in providing services. The LINk was still being established and, in common with other sites, it was proving difficult for the LINk to engage with social services. The worsening financial climate had encouraged more emphasis on the return on investment for public health interventions and promoted greater integration across health and social care. Methods for prioritisation were being developed and programme budgeting was being used to aid disinvestment.

Site 10 was the result of a complex reorganisation, and was made up of former PCTs with different levels of resource and performance. It related to a two-tier authority and had the largest population of the case study sites, a greater than average population of older people and better health than average for England. The DPH was a joint appointment with the county council and produced a joint public health report. There were good working relationships with the local authority, a joint strategic plan with the county council, jointly funded posts and joint health and social care teams. The DPH report focused on equity of service provision, informed by benchmarking data. The PCT's financial commitment to improving health included a 5% shift of resources over the next five years but this was reliant on growth funding. The JSNA was locality based and involved widespread canvassing of community views, the VCS and PBC, and was tied in to locality commissioning arrangements with PBC, with senior public health staff working at locality level. It had demonstrated variation, resulting in priority communities being identified. PBC had progressed slowly: insufficient PCT funds to allow practices to reinvest savings had meant that practices had lost interest. Some considered the move to PCTs from primary care groups had led to the loss of multidisciplinary, locality-based commissioning. Governance issues in PBC were considered difficult to resolve and there was frustration over the imposition of central priorities. Methods for public consultation were well developed. Board meetings were held in public across the county. The LINk had been slow to become established and representativeness was an issue. Ethical frameworks for decision making had been developed. However, more demanding targets in relation to acute care had led to reduced resources for preventive services.

Note

[1] The full report and details of the project team can be found at: www.nets.nihr.ac.uk/projects/hsdr/081716208

References

Abbott, S.J. (2006) *Primary care-led commissioning in England and Wales*, ESRC Full Research Report, RES-000-22-1198. Swindon: ESRC.

Acheson, D. (1988) *Public health in England: The report of the committee of inquiry into the future development of the public health function*, London: HMSO.

Acheson, D. (chair) (1998) *Independent inquiry into inequalities in health*, London: The Stationery Office.

Airoldi, M., Morton, A., Smith, J. and Bevan, G. (2011) *Healthcare prioritisation at the local level: a socio-technical approach. Priority-setting for population health*, Working paper No. 7, Department of Management, London School of Economics (www.lse.ac.uk/management/documents/WP7_-_Healthcare_prioritisation_at_the_local_level_A_socio-technical_approach.pdf).

Appleby, J., Harrison, T., Hawkins, L. and Dixon, A. (2012) *Payment by results: How can payment systems help to deliver better care?* London: King's Fund.

Arnstein, S.R. (1969) 'A ladder of citizen participation', *Journal of the American Institute of Planners*, vol. 35, pp. 216–24.

Association of Public Health Observatories and Department of Health (n.d.) *Health inequalities intervention toolkit*, London Health Observatory (www.lho.org.uk/LHO_Topics/Analytic_Tools/HealthInequalitiesInterventionToolkit.aspx; 2010).

Audit Commission (2003) *Corporate governance: Improvement and trust in local public services*, London: Audit Commission.

Audit Commission (2005) *Governing partnerships: Bridging the accountability gap*, London: Audit Commission.

Audit Commission (2007) *A prescription for partnership: Engaging clinicians in financial management*, London: Audit Commission.

Audit Commission (2009a) *Working better together? Managing local strategic partnerships*, London: Audit Commission.

Audit Commission (2009b) *Payment by results data assurance framework 2008/09: Key messages from Year 2 of the national clinical coding audit programme*, London: Audit Commission.

Audit Commission (2010) *Healthy balance: A review of public health performance and spending*, Health Briefing, March, London: Audit Commission.

Barnes, M., Skelcher, C., Beirens, H., Dalziel, R., Jeffares, S. and Wilson, L. (2008) *Designing citizen centred governance*, York: Joseph Rowntree Foundation.

Bennett, B., Gostin, L., Magnusson, R. and Martin, R. (2009) 'Health governance: law, regulation and policy', *Public Health*, vol. 123, pp. 207–12.

Bentley, C. (2008) *Systematically addressing health inequalities*, National support team for health inequalities, London: Department of Health.

Bernstein, H., Cosford, P. and Williams, A. (2010) *Enabling effective delivery of health and wellbeing: An independent report* (http://base-uk.org/sites/base-uk.org/files/%5Buser-raw%5D/11-06/pc.pdf).

Bevan, G. and Hood, C. (2006) 'Have targets improved performance in the English NHS?' *British Medical Journal*, vol. 332, pp. 419–22.

Black, D. (1980) *Inequalities in health: Report of a research working group*, Chaired by Sir Douglas Black (The Black Report), London: DHSS (www.sochealth.co.uk/public-health-and-wellbeing/poverty-and-inequality/the-black-report-1980/).

Blackman, T., Greene, A., Hunter, D.J., McKee, L., Elliott, E., Harrington, B., Marks, L. and Williams, G. (2006) 'Performance assessment and wicked problems: the case of health inequalities', *Public Policy and Administration*, vol. 21, no. 2, pp. 66–80.

Blackman, T., Harrington, B., Elliott, E., Greene, A., Hunter, D.J., Marks, L., McKee, L. and Williams, G. (2012) 'Framing health inequalities for local intervention: comparative case studies', *Sociology of Health and Illness*, vol. 34, no. 1, pp. 49–63.

Blagescu, M., Las Casas, L. de and Lloyd, R. (2005) *Pathways to accountability: The GAP framework*, London: One World Trust.

Bovens, M. (2010) 'Two concepts of accountability: accountability as a virtue and as a mechanism', *West European Politics*, vol. 33, no. 5, pp. 946–67.

British Academy (2014) *'If you could do one thing …'. Nine local actions to reduce health inequalities*, London: The British Academy.

Brock, D.W. (2007) 'Ethical issues in applying quantitative models for setting priorities in prevention', ch. 7 in Dawson, A. and Verweij, M. (eds) *Ethics, prevention and public health*, Oxford: Oxford University Press.

Brotherton, P. and Battersby, J. (2011) *Joint Strategic Needs Assessment: Data inventory*, London: Local Government Group.

Butland, B., Jebb, S., Kopelman, P., McPherson, K., Thomas, S., Mardell, J. and Parry, V. (2007) *Tackling obesities: Future choices*. Project report, Government Office for Science, London: Department of Innovation Universities and Skills.

Campbell, F. and Heron, C. (2010) *Commissioning for health: A guide for overview and scrutiny committees on NHS commissioning and the world class commissioning programme*, London: Centre for Public Scrutiny.

Campbell, S.M., Reeves, D., Kontopantelis, E., Sibbald, B. and Roland, M. (2009) 'Effects of pay for performance on the quality of primary care in England', *New England Journal of Medicine*, vol. 361, pp. 368–78.

Capewell, S., Allender, S., Critchley, J., Lloyd-Williams, F., O'Flaherty, M., Rayner, M. and Scarborough, P. (2008) *Modelling the UK burden of cardiovascular disease to 2020: A research report for the cardio and vascular coalition and the British Heart Foundation*, London: British Heart Foundation.

Care Quality Commission (2013) *Raising standards, putting people first – our strategy for 2013 to 2016*, Newcastle upon Tyne: Care Quality Commission (www.cqc.org.uk/sites/default/files/media/documents/20130503_cqc_strategy_2013_final_cm_tagged.pdf).

Checkland, K., Allen, P., Coleman, A., Segar, J., McDermott, I., Harrison, S., Petsoulas, C. and Peckham, S. (2013) 'Accountable to whom, for what? An exploration of the early development of Clinical Commissioning Groups in the English NHS', *BMJ Open*,
vol. 3: e003769. doi:10.1136/bmjopen-2013-003769.

Christianson, J., Leatherman, S. and Sutherland, K. (2009) *Financial incentives, healthcare providers and quality improvements: A review of the evidence*, London: The Health Foundation.

Claxton, K., Sculpher, M. and Culyer, T. (2007) *Mark versus Luke? Appropriate methods for the evaluation of public health interventions*, CHE research paper 31, York: Centre for Health Economics, University of York.

Coleman, A. and Harrison, S. (2006) *The implementation of local authority scrutiny of primary health care 2002–5*, Manchester: National Primary Care Research and Development Centre.

Coleman, A., Checkland, K. and Harrison, S. (2009) 'Still puzzling: patient and public involvement in commissioning', *Journal of Integrated Care*, vol. 17, no. 6, pp. 23–30.

Coleman, A., Checkland, K., McDermott, I. and Harrison, S. (2011) 'Patient and public involvement in the restructured NHS', *Journal of Integrated Care*, vol. 19, no. 4, pp. 30 6.

Committee on Standards in Public Life (1995) *Standards in public life: First report of the Committee on Standards in Public Life*, Cm. 2850, London: The Stationery Office.

Cooke, G. and Muir, R. (2012) *The relational state*, London: Institute for Public Policy Research.

Courpasson, D. (2000) 'Managerial strategies of domination: power in soft bureaucracies', *Organization Studies*, vol. 21, no. 1, pp. 141–61.

Crump, H. (2009) 'World class commissioning table: PCTs exceed expectations in year one', *Health Service Journal*, 5 March.

Curry, N., Goodwin, N., Naylor, C. and Robertson, R. (2008) *Practice-based commissioning: Reinvigorate, replace or abandon?* London: King's Fund.

Davies, C., Anand, P., Artigas, L., Holloway, J., McConway, K., Newman, J., Storey, J. and Thompson, G. (2005) *Links between governance, incentives and outcomes: A review of the literature*, London: National Co-ordinating Centre for NHS Service Delivery and Organisation R&D (NCCSDO).

Davies, J.S. (2011) *Challenging governance theory: From network to hegemony*, Bristol: The Policy Press.

Davies, R., Normand, C., Raftery, J., Roderick, P. and Sanderson, C. (2004) *Policy analysis for coronary heart disease: A simulation model of interventions, costs and outcomes*, London: Department of Health.

Dawson, A. and Verweij, M. (eds) (2007) *Ethics, prevention and public health*, Oxford: Oxford University Press.

Department for Communities and Local Government (2007) *The new performance framework for local authorities and local authority partnerships: Single set of national indicators*, London: Department for Communities and Local Government.

Department of Health (2003a) *Tackling health inequalities: A programme for action*, Cm 6374, London: Department of Health.

Department of Health (2003b) *Overview and Scrutiny of Health – Guidance*, London: Department of Health.

Department of Health (2004) *National standards, local action: Health and social care standards and planning framework 2005/06–2007/8*, London: Department of Health.

Department of Health (2005) *Commissioning a patient-led NHS*, Cm 6268, London: Department of Health.

Department of Health (2006a) *PCT and SHA roles and functions*, London: Department of Health.

Department of Health (2006b) *A stronger local voice: A framework for creating a stronger local voice in the development of health and social care services*, London: Department of Health.

Department of Health (2007a) *Commissioning framework for health and well-being*, London: Department of Health.

Department of Health (2007b) *World class commissioning: Vision*, London: Department of Health.

Department of Health (2007c) *World class commissioning: Competencies*, London: Department of Health.

Department of Health (2007d) *Guidance on Joint Strategic Needs Assessment*, London: Department of Health.

Department of Health (2007e) *Options for the future of payment by results: 2008/09 to 2010/11*, Leeds: Department of Health.

Department of Health (2008a) *Commissioning assurance handbook*, London: Department of Health.

Department of Health (2008b) *Healthy weight, healthy lives: A cross-government strategy for England*, London: Department of Health.

Department of Health (2008c) *The NHS in England: The operating framework for 2009/10*, London: Department of Health.

Department of Health (2008d) *Real involvement: Working with people to improve health services: Guidance for NHS organisations on section 242(1B) of the NHS Act 2006, the duty to involve and good involvement practice*, London: Department of Health.

Department of Health (2008e) *Local Involvement Networks explained*, London: Department of Health.

Department of Health (2009a) *World class commissioning assurance handbook Year 2*, London: Department of Health.

Department of Health (2009b) *Transforming community services: Enabling new patterns of provision*, London: Department of Health.

Department of Health/NHS Finance Performance and Operations (2009c) *The operating framework for 2010/11 for the NHS in England*, London: Department of Health.

Department of Health (2009d) *The statement of NHS accountability*, London: Department of Health.

Department of Health (2011a) *Public health in local government: Commissioning responsibilities*, London: Department of Health.

Department of Health (2011b) *Public health in local government: Public health advice to NHS commissioners*, London: Department of Health.

Department of Health (2011c) *Developing clinical commissioning groups: Towards authorisation*, London: Department of Health.

Department of Health (2011d) *Healthy lives, healthy people: A tobacco control plan for England*, London: Department of Health.

Department of Health (2011e) *Healthy lives healthy people: A call to action on obesity in England*, London: Department of Health.

Department of Health (2012a) *Improving outcomes and supporting transparency, Part 1A: A public health outcomes framework for England, 2013–2016*, London. Department of Health.

Department of Health (2012b) *The NHS Outcomes Framework 2013/14*, London: Department of Health.

Department of Health (2012c) *The Adult Social Care Outcomes Framework, 2013/2016*, London: Department of Health

Department of Health (2012d) *Healthy lives, healthy people: Update on public health funding*, London: Department of Health.

Department of Health (2013a) *Statutory guidance on Joint Strategic Needs Assessments and Joint Health and Wellbeing Strategies*, London: Department of Health.

Department of Health (2013b) *The NHS Constitution for England*, London: Department of Health.

Department of Health (2013c) *Guide to the healthcare system in England: Including the statement of NHS accountability*, London: Department of Health.

Dixon, A., Khachatryan, A., Wallace, A., Peckham, S., Boyce, T. and Gillam, S. (2010) *The Quality and Outcomes Framework: Does it reduce health inequalities?* Final report. NIHR Service Delivery and Organisation Programme.

Doran, T., Fullwood, C., Kontopantelis, E. and Reeves, D. (2008) 'Effect of financial incentives on inequalities in the delivery of primary clinical care in England: analysis of clinical activity indicators for the quality and outcomes framework', *The Lancet*, vol. 372, pp. 728–36.

Drummond, M., Weatherly, H., Claxton, K., Cookson, R., Ferguson, B., Godfrey, C., Rice, N., Sculpher, M. and Sowden, A. (2007) *Assessing the challenges of applying standard methods of economic evaluation*, York: Public Health Research Consortium.

Drummond, M., Weatherly, H., Ferguson, B. (2008) 'Economic evaluation of health interventions', *British Medical Journal*, vol. 337, p. a1204.

Exworthy, M., Powell, M. and Mohan J. (1999) 'The NHS: quasi-market, quasi-hierarchy and quasi-network?' *Public Money and Management*, vol. 19, no. 4, pp. 15–22.

Farrar, S., Sussex, J., Yi, D., Sutton, M., Chalkley, M., Scott, A., Sutton, M. and Yuen, P. (2007) *National evaluation of payment by results*, Aberdeen: University of Aberdeen.

Fleetcroft, R., Steel, N., Cookson, R., Walker, S. and Howe, A. (2012) 'Incentive payments are not related to expected health gain in the pay for performance scheme for UK primary care: cross-sectional analysis', *BMC Health Services Research*, vol. 12, no. 94.

Flynn, R. (2004) '"Soft bureaucracy", governmentality and clinical governance: theoretical approaches to emergent policy', ch. 2 in Gray, A. and Harrison, S. (eds) *Governing medicine: Theory and practice*, Maidenhead: Open University Press, 11–27.

Foot, J. and Hopkins, T. (2010) *A glass half-full: How an asset approach can improve community health and well-being*, Improvement and Development Agency, London: Local Government Association.

Fox-Rushby, J., Boehler, C., Hanney, S., Roberts, I., Beresford, P. and Buxton, M. (2008) *Prioritisation of preventive services: Determining the applicability of research from the US to the English context*. Final report commissioned for Health England by the Department of Health Policy Research Programme, Brunel University: Health Economics Research Group.

Francis Inquiry (2010) *Independent inquiry into care provided by Mid Staffordshire NHS Foundation Trust January 2005–March 2009*, vol. 1, Chaired by Robert Francis QC, London: The Stationery Office.

Francis Inquiry (2013) *Report of the Mid Staffordshire NHS Foundation Trust Public Inquiry*, Chaired by Robert Francis QC, London: The Stationery Office.

Frenk, J. and Moon, S. (2013) 'Governance challenges in global health', *New England Journal of Medicine*, vol. 368, pp. 936–42.

Frosini, F., Dixon, A. and Roberston, R. (2012) 'Competition in the NHS: a provider perspective', *Journal of Health Services Research and Policy*, vol. 17 (suppl. 1), pp. 16–22.

Fuerth, L.S. (2009) 'Foresight and anticipatory governance', *Foresight*, vol. 11, no. 4, pp. 14–32.

Galbraith-Emami, S. (2013) *Public health law and non-communicable diseases*, London: UK Health Forum.

Gash, T., Hallsworth, M., Ismail, S. and Paun, A. (2008) *Performance art: Enabling better management in the public services*, London: Institute for Government.

Glasby, J. (ed.) (2012) *Commissioning for health and well-being: An introduction*, Bristol: The Policy Press.

Glasby, J. and Dickinson, H. (2014) *Partnership working in health and social care: What is integrated care and how can we deliver it?* (2nd edn), Bristol: The Policy Press.

Goddard, M., Mannion, R. and Smith, P. (2000) 'Enhancing performance in health care: a theoretical perspective on agency and the role of information', *Health Economics*, vol. 9, pp. 95–107.

Goodwin, N., Perri 6, Peck, E., Freeman, T. and Posaner, R. (2004) *Managing across diverse networks: Lessons from other sectors*, Birmingham: University of Birmingham, Health Services Management Centre.

Gosden, T. and Torgerson, D. (1997) 'The effect of fundholding on prescribing and referral costs: a review of the evidence', *Health Policy*, vol. 40, pp. 103–14.

Gostin, L.O. (2008) *Public health law: Power, duty, restraint* (2nd edn), Berkeley: University of California Press.

Gostin, L.O. and Stone, L. (2007) 'Health of the people: the highest law?', ch. 2 in Dawson, A. and Verweij, M. (eds) *Ethics, prevention and public health*, Oxford: Oxford University Press.

Graham, H. (2009) 'Health inequalities, social determinants and public health policy', *Policy and Politics*, vol. 37, no. 4, pp. 463–79.

Graham, H. (2010) 'Where is the future in public health?' *The Milbank Quarterly*, vol. 88, no. 2, pp. 149–68.

Graham, J., Amos, B. and Plumptre, T. (2003) *Principles of good governance in the 21st century*, Ottawa: Institute on Governance.

Gray, A. (2004) 'Governing medicine: an introduction', ch. 1 in Gray, A. and Harrison, S.R. (eds) *Governing medicine*, Maidenhead: Open University Press.

Guindo, L.A., Wagner, M., Baltussen, R., Rindress, D., Van Til, J., Kind, P. and Goetghebeur, M.M. (2012) 'From efficacy to equity: literature review of decision criteria for resource allocation and healthcare decision making', *Cost Effectiveness and Resource Allocation*, vol. 10, no. 9.

Hacking, J.M., Muller, S. and Buchan, I.E. (2011) 'Trends in mortality from 1965 to 2008 across the English north–south divide: comparative observational study', *British Medical Journal* 342: d508.

Hallsworth, M. (2011) *System stewardship: The future of policy making?* Working paper, London: Institute for Government.

Ham, C. (2007) *Clinically integrated systems: The next step in English health reform*, London: The Nuffield Trust.

Hanlon, P.W. and Carlisle, S. (2008) 'Do we face a third revolution in human history? If so, how will public health respond?' *Journal of Public Health*, vol. 30, pp. 355–61.

Hanlon, P., Carlisle, S., Reilly, D. and Lyon, A. (2011) 'Making the case for a "fifth wave" in public health', *Public Health*, vol. 125, no. 1, pp. 30–6.

Harding, E., Kane, M., Shaw, L., Gamsu, M. and Whyte, D. (2011) *Joint strategic needs assessment: A springboard for action*, London: Local Government Improvement and Development Healthy Communities Programme.

Harrison, D., Ziglio, E., Levin. L. and Morgan, A. (2004) *Assets for health and development: Developing a conceptual framework*, European Office for Investment for Health and Development, Venice: World Health Organization.

Harrison, S., Dowswell, G. and Milewa, T. (2002) 'Guest editorial: public and user involvement in the UK National Health Service', *Health and Social Care in the Community*, vol. 10, no. 2, pp. 63–6.

Health and Social Care Information Centre (2013) *Investment in General Practice, England, Wales, Northern Ireland and Scotland – 2008–09 to 2012–13*.

Healthcare Commission (2007a) *No ifs, no buts: Improving services for tobacco control*, London: Healthcare Commission.

Healthcare Commission (2007b) *Managing diabetes: Improving services for people with diabetes*, London: Healthcare Commission.

Healthcare Commission (2007c) *Performing better: A focus on sexual health services in England*, London: Healthcare Commission.

Healthcare Commission and Audit Commission (2008) *Are we choosing health? The impact of policy on health improvement programmes and services*, London: Commission for Healthcare Audit and Inspection.

Health England (Expert Advisory Panel on Preventative Health Spending) (2007) *Definitions and measures of preventative health spending*, Report no. 1, Oxford: Health England.

Health England (Expert Advisory Panel on Preventative Health Spending) (2009) *Prevention and preventative spending*, Oxford: Health England.

Healthwatch England (2013) *Annual Report 2012/13*, Newcastle upon Tyne: Healthwatch England.

HM Government (2010a) *The Coalition: our programme for government*, Cabinet Office, London: 2010.

HM Government (2010b) *Decentralisation and the Localism Bill: An essential guide*, London: Department for Communities and Local Government (https://www.gov.uk/government/uploads/system/uploads/attachment_data/file/5951/1793908.pdf).

HM Treasury (2007a) *PSA Delivery 18: Promote better health and wellbeing for all*, London: The Stationery Office.

HM Treasury (2007b) *Pre-budget report and comprehensive spending review*, London: The Stationery Office.

HM Treasury and Department for Communities and Local Government (2010) *Total place: A whole area approach to public services*, London: HM Treasury.

Hood, C. (2006) 'Gaming in targetworld: the targets approach to managing British public services', *Public Administration Review*, vol. 66, no. 4, pp. 515–21.

Hood, C. (2010) 'Accountability and transparency: Siamese twins, matching parts, awkward couple?' *West European Politics*, vol. 33, no. 5, pp. 989–1009.

Hooghe, L. and Marks, G. (2001) 'Types of multi-level governance', *European Integration online Papers* (EIoP), vol. 5, no. 11.

House of Commons Health Committee (2007) *Patient and public involvement in the NHS*, Third Report of Session 2006–07, vol. 1, HC 278-I, London: The Stationery Office.

House of Commons Health Committee (2009) *Health inequalities*, Third Report of Session 2008–09, vol. 1, HC 286-1, London: The Stationery Office.

House of Commons Health Committee (2010) *Commissioning*, Fourth Report of Session 2009–10, vol. 1, HC 268-I, London: The Stationery Office.

House of Commons Health Committee (2011) *Commissioning*, Third Report of Session 2010–11, HC 513-1, London: The Stationery Office.

House of Commons Communities and Local Government Committee (2013) *The role of local authorities in health issues*, Eighth Report of Session 2012–13, vol. 1, HC 694, London: The Stationery Office.

Humphries, R. and Galea, A. (2013) *Health and wellbeing boards, one year on*, London: King's Fund.

Hunter, D.J. (2013) *To Market! To Market!* Centre for Health and the Public Interest. (http://chpi.org.uk/wp-content/uploads/2013/07/David-Hunter-to-market-to-market pdf)

Hunter, D.J. and Marks, L. (2005) *Managing for health: What incentives exist for NHS managers to focus on wider health issues?* London: King's Fund.

Hunter, D.J., Marks, L. and Smith, K.E. (2010) *The public health system in England*, Bristol: The Policy Press.

Hunter, D.J. and Perkins, N. (2014) *Partnership working in public health*, Bristol: The Policy Press.

Hunter, D.J., Popay, J., Tannahill, C., Whitehead, M. and Elson, T. (2009) *Cross-cutting sub-group report: Learning lessons from the past: shaping a different future*, London: UCL Institute of Health Equity, Marmot Review Working Committee 3.

Improvement and Development Agency (2007) *A very English revolution: Delivering bolder and better local area agreements*, London: Local Government Association.

Independent Commission on Good Governance in Public Services (2004) *The good governance standard for public services*, London: Office for Public Management, Chartered Institute of Public Finance and Accountability.

Inglis, J. (2012) *Guide to commissioning for maximum value*, Social Return on Investment Network, London: Local Government Association.

Institute of Medicine (2002) *The future of the public's health in the 21st century*, Washington, DC: Institute of Medicine.

Jochelson, K. (2005) *Nanny or steward? The role of local government in public health*, London: King's Fund.

Jochum, V., Pratten, B. and Wilding, K. (2005) *Civil renewal and active citizenship: A guide to the debate*, London: NCVO.

Joffe, M. and Mindell, J. (2005) 'Health impact assessment', *Occupational and Environmental Medicine*, vol. 62, pp. 907–12.

Kahneman, D. and Tversky, A. (1979) 'Prospect theory: an analysis of decision under risk', *Econometrica*, XLVII, pp. 263–91.

Kane, R.L., Johnson, P.E., Town, R.J. and Butler, M. (2004) 'Economic incentives for preventive care: evidence report', *Technology Assessment*, no. 101, pp. 1–141.

Kass, N.E. (2001) 'An ethics framework for public health', *American Journal of Public Health*, vol. 91, no. 11, pp. 176–82.

Kass, N.E. (2004) 'Public health ethics: from foundations and frameworks to justice and global public health', *Journal of Law, Medicine and Ethics*, vol. 32, pp. 232–42.

Kelly, M.P., McDaid, D., Ludbrook, A. and Powell, J. (2005) *Economic appraisal of public health interventions: Briefing paper*, London: Health Development Agency.

Kelly, M., Stewart, E., Morgan, A., Killoran, A., Fischer, A., Threlfall, A. and Bonnefoy, J. (2009) 'A conceptual framework for public health: NICE's emerging approach', *Public Health*, vol. 123, no. 1, pp. e14–e20.

Kemm, J. and Parry, J. (2004) 'What is HIA? Introduction and overview', in Kemm, J., Parry, J. and Palmer, S. (eds) *Health impact assessment: Concepts, theory, techniques and applications*, Oxford: Oxford University Press, pp. 1–14.

Kickbusch, I. and Gleicher, D. (2012) *Governance for health in the 21st century*, Copenhagen: WHO Regional Office for Europe.

King's Fund (n.d.) 'Have targets improved NHS performance?' (www.kingsfund.org.uk/projects/general-election-2010/key-election-questions/performance-targets).

Lalonde, M. (1974) *A new perspective on the health of Canadians*, Ottawa: Government of Canada.

Langdown, C. and Peckham, S. (2013) 'The use of financial incentives to help improve health outcomes: is the quality and outcomes framework fit for purpose? A systematic review', *Journal of Public Health*, doi: 10.1093/pubmed/fdt077. First published online: 8 August 2013.

Le Grand, J. (2003) *Motivation, agency, and public policy: Of knights and knaves, pawns and queens*, Oxford: Oxford University Press.

Le Grand, J., Titmuss, R. and Srivastava, D. (2009) *Incentives for prevention*, Health England Report No. 3.

Leary, S. and Palmer, M. (2009) 'A healthy option', *Healthcare Finance*, vol. 29, pp. 31–2.

Lewis, G., Curry, N. and Bardsley, M. (2011) *Choosing a predictive risk model: A guide for commissioners in England*, London: Nuffield Trust.

Lipsky, M. (1980) *Street-level bureaucracy: Dilemmas of the individual in public services*, New York: Russell Sage Foundation.

Local Government Association (2012) *Commissioning for better public services*, London: Local Government Association.

Local Government Association (2013) *Delivering effective local healthwatch: Key success features*, London: Local Government Association.

Local Government Association (2014) *Public health transformation, nine months on: Bedding in and reaching out*, London: Local Government Association.

Longley, M., Riley, N., Davies, P. and Hernández-Quevedo, C. (2012) 'United Kingdom (Wales): health system review', *Health Systems in Transition*, vol. 14, no. 11, pp. 1–84.

Lundgren, B. (2009) 'Experiences from the Swedish determinants-based public health policy', *International Journal of Health Services*, vol. 39, no. 3, pp. 491–507.

Maciosek, M.V., Coffield, A.B., Edwards, N.M., Flottemesch, T.J., Goodman, M.J. and Solberg, L.I. (2006) 'Priorities among effective clinical preventive services: results of a systematic review and analysis', *American Journal of Preventive Medicine*, vol., 31, pp. 52–61.

Mackenbach, J.P. (2010) 'Has the English strategy to reduce health inequalities failed?' *Social Science & Medicine*, vol. 71, pp. 1249–53.

Maguire, K. and Truscott, F. (2006) *Active governance: The value added by community involvement in governance through local strategic partnerships*, York: Joseph Rowntree Foundation.

Mannion, R. and Davies, H.T.O. (2008) 'Incentives in health systems; developing theory, investigating practice', *Journal of Health Organization and Management*, vol 22, no 1, pp 5–10.

Mannion, R., Davies, H.T. and Marshall, M. (2003) *Cultures for performance in health care: Evidence of the relationship between organisational culture and organisational performance in the NHS*, York: York Centre for Health Economics.

Mannion, R., Marini, G. and Street, A. (2008) 'Implementing payment by results in the English NHS. Changing incentives and the role of information', *Journal of Health Organization and Management*, vol 22, no 1, pp 79–88.

Marini, G. and Street, A. (2007) 'A transaction costs analysis of changing contractual relations in the English NHS', *Health Policy*, vol. 83, pp. 17–26.

Marks L. (2007) 'Fault lines between policy and practice in local partnerships', *Journal of Health Organization and Management*, vol. 21, no. 2, pp. 136–48.

Marks, L. (in press) 'Explanatory note on accountability for social determinants of health equity', in Brown, C. et al. *Governance for social determinants and equity in health. Companion resource guide: Main principles, current trends and promising practices.* Copenhagen: WHO Regional Office for Europe.

Marks, L. and Hunter, D.J. (2005) 'Moving upstream or muddying the waters? Incentives for managing for health', *Public Health*, vol. 119, pp. 974–80.

Marks, L., Brown, J., Jennings-Peel, H. and Hunter, D.J. (2007) *Guidance for the NHS and other sectors on interventions that reduce the rates of premature death in disadvantaged areas: Proactive case finding and retention and improving access to services: Mapping review*, London: NICE.

Marks, L., Cave, S. and Hunter, D.J. (2010) 'Public health governance: views of key stakeholders', *Public Health*, vol. 124, pp. 55–59.

Marks, L., Cave, S., Hunter, D.J., Mason, J., Peckham, S., Wallace, A., Mason, A., Weatherly, H. and Melvin, K. (2011a) *Public health governance and primary care delivery: A triangulated study*, Final report, NIHR Service Delivery and Organisation programme (www.nets.nihr.ac.uk/projects/hsdr/081716208).

Marks, L., Hunter, D.J. and Alderslade, R. (2011b) *Strengthening public health capacity and services in Europe: A concept note*, Copenhagen: WHO Regional Office for Europe and Durham University.

Marks, L., Cave, S., Hunter, D.J., Mason, J., Peckham, S. and Wallace, A. (2011c) 'Governance for health and well-being in the English NHS', *Journal of Health Services Research and Policy*, vol. 16 (suppl. 1), pp. 14–21.

Marks, L., Cave, S., Wallace, A., Mason, A., Hunter, D.J., Mason, J. and Peckham, S. (2011d) 'Incentivizing preventive services in primary care: perspectives on local enhanced services', *Journal of Public Health*, vol. 33, no. 4, pp. 556–64.

Marks, L., Weatherly, H. and Mason, A. (2013a) 'Prioritising investment in public health and health equity: what can commissioners do?' *Public Health*, vol. 127, no. 5, pp. 410–18.

Marks, L., Ormston, C., Hunter, D.J., Thokala, P., Payne, N., Salway, S., Vale, L., Gray, J. and McCafferty, S. (2013b) *Prioritising public health intervention in local authorities: A scoping study of approaches for decision-support* (www.fuse.ac.uk/shifting-the-gravity-of-spending%3F-).

Marmot, M. (Chair), UCL Institute of Health Equity (2013) *Review of social determinants and the health divide in the WHO European region: Final report*, Copenhagen: WHO Regional Office for Europe.

Marmot, M., Allen, J., Bell, R., Bloomer, E. and Goldblatt, P. (2012) 'WHO European review of social determinants of health and the health divide', *The Lancet*, vol. 380, pp. 1011–29.

Marmot Review (2010) *Fair society, healthy lives: Strategic review of health inequalities in England post-2010*, London: The Marmot Review.

Marshall, T. and Hothersall, E. (2012) 'Needs assessment', ch. 2 in Glasby, J. (ed.) *Commissioning for health and well being*, Bristol: The Policy Press, 43–62.

Martuzzi, M. and Tickner, J.A. (eds) (2004) *The precautionary principle: Protecting public health, the environment and the future of our children*, Copenhagen: WHO Regional Office for Europe.

Matrix Insight (2009a) *Valuing health: Developing a business case for health improvement, Final report*, London: Improvement and Development Agency.

Matrix Insight (2009b) *Prioritising investments in preventative health: Project undertaken for Health England, the national reference group for health and wellbeing*, London: Matrix Insight (http://help.matrixknowledge.com/).

Matrix Insight (2011) *Business case for health and well being*, Final Report, Commissioned by the Local Government Association, London: Matrix Insight.

Maybin, J., Addicott, R., Dixon, A. and Storey, J. (2011) *Accountability in the NHS: Implications of the government's reform programme*, London: King's Fund.

Mays, N. (2013) 'Evaluating the Labour government's English NHS health system reforms: the 2008 Darzi reforms', Editorial, *Journal of Health Services Research and Policy*, vol. 18, no. 2 (suppl.), pp. 1–10.

Mays, N., Goodwin, N., Bevan, G. and Wyke, S. (1997) 'What is total purchasing?' *British Medical Journal*, vol. 315, p. 652.

Mays, N. and Tan, S. (2012) 'Evaluating Labour's market reforms 2002-10', *Journal of Health Services Research and Policy*, vol 17 (Suppl 1), pp. 1–6.

McCafferty, S., Williams, I., Hunter, D.J., Robinson, S., Donaldson, C. and Bate, A. (2012) 'Implementing world class commissioning competencies', *Journal of Health Services Research and Policy*, vol. 17, pp. 40–8.

McDaid, D. and Needle, J. (2008) 'What use has been made of economic evaluation in public health? A systematic review of the literature', in Dawson, S. and Morris, Z.S. (eds) *Future public health: Burdens, challenges and opportunities*, Basingstoke: Palgrave Macmillan.

McDonald, R., Harrison, S. and Checkland, K. (2008) 'Incentives and control in primary health care: findings from English pay-for-performance case studies', *Journal of Health Organization and Management*, vol. 22, no. 1, pp. 48–62.

McDonald, R., Cheraghi-Sohi, S., Tickle, M., Roland, M., Doran, T., Campbell, S., Ashcroft, D., Sanders, C., Harrison, S., Mannion, R. and Milsom, K. (2010) *The impact of incentives on the behaviour and performance of primary care professionals*, Final report, NIHR Service Delivery and Organisation Programme (www.sdo.nihr.ac.uk/files/project/158-final-report.pdf).

McDonald, R., Zaidi, S., Todd, S., Konteh, F., Hussain, K., Brown, S., Kristensen, S.R. and Sutton, M. (2013) *Evaluation of the Commissioning for Quality and Innovation framework*, Final report, Nottingham: University of Nottingham.

McMichael, A.J., Woodruff, R.E. and Hales, S. (2006) 'Climate change and human health: present and future risks', *The Lancet*, vol. 367, pp. 859–69.

Melvin, K. (2010) *Evaluation of Tower Hamlets Involvement Network*, Final report. Commissioned by Tower Hamlets Involvement Network.

Merkur, S., Sassi, F. and McDaid, D. (2013) *Promoting health, preventing disease: Is there an economic case?* Policy report 6, Copenhagen: World Health Organization.

Michaelson, J., Mahony, S. and Schifferes, J. (2012) *Measuring well-being: A guide for practitioners*, London: New Economics Foundation (http://dnwssx4l7gl7s. cloudfront.net/nefoundation/default/page/-/files/Measuring_well-being_ handbook_FINAL.pdf).

Milgrom, P. and Roberts, J. (1992) *Economics, organization and management*, Englewood Cliffs, NJ: Prentice Hall.

Millar, R., Powell, M. and Dixon, A. (2012) 'What was the programme theory of New Labour's health system reforms?' *Journal of Health Services Research and Policy*, vol. 17 (suppl. 1), pp. 7–15.

Millett, C., Gray, J., Saxena, S. and Majeed, A. (2007) 'Impact of a pay-for-performance incentive on support for smoking cessation and on smoking prevalence among people with diabetes', *Canadian Medical Association Journal*, vol. 176, pp. 1705–10.

Milton, B., Moonan, M., Taylor-Robinson, D. and Whitehead, M. (eds) (2010) *How can the health equity impact of universal policies be evaluated? Insights into approaches and next steps*, Copenhagen: WHO Regional Office for Europe and University of Liverpool.

Ministry of Health and Care Services (2011) *The Norwegian Public Health Act, 2011* (www.regjeringen.no/upload/HOD/Hoeringer%20FHA_FOS/123. pdf).

Ministry of Social Affairs and Health (2008) *National action plan to reduce health inequalities 2008–2011*, Helsinki: Ministry of Social Affairs and Health, Finland. (http://pre20090115.stm.fi/pr1227003636140/passthru.pdf).

Morgan, A., Ellis, S., Field, J., Owen, L., Jones, D., Minchin, M., McArthur, C., Doohan, E., Hodgson, G. and Pickard, L. (2011) *Supporting investment in public health: Review of methods for assessing cost effectiveness, cost impact and return on investment. Proof of concept report*, London: NICE.

Murphy, L. and Turner, S. (2012) *Local healthwatch, health and wellbeing boards and health scrutiny*, London: Centre for Public Scrutiny.

Murray, C.J.L., Richards, M.A., Newton, J.M. et al. (2013) 'UK health performance: findings of the Global Burden of Disease study 2010', *The Lancet*, vol. 381, pp. 997–1020.

Newman, J. (2001) *Modernising governance: New Labour policy and society*. London: Sage.

NHS Commissioning Board (2013) *Commissioning for quality and innovation* (www.england.nhs.uk/wp-content/uploads/2013/02/cquin-guidance.pdf).

NHS Confederation (2011a) *The Joint Strategic Needs Assessment: A vital tool to guide commissioning*, London: NHS Confederation in association with Local Government Improvement and Development and the Royal Society for Public Health.

NHS Confederation (2011b) *Patient and public engagement in the new commissioning system. Discussion paper*, London: The NHS Confederation.

NHS Confederation (2012) *Making a local difference: State of play and challenges ahead for health and wellbeing boards*, London: The NHS Confederation.

NHS Confederation Primary Care Trust Network (2011) *The legacy of Primary Care Trusts*, London: The NHS Confederation.

NHS Employers (2013) *2013/14 General Medical Services (GMS) contract quality and outcomes framework* (www.nhsemployers.org/your-workforce/primary-care-contacts/general-medical-services/quality-and-outcomes-framework).

NHS England (2013) *Quality Premium 2013/14 guidance for GPs* (www.england.nhs.uk/wp-content/uploads/2013/05/qual-premium.pdf).

NHS England (2014) *Everyone counts: Planning for patients 2014/15–2018/19*, London: NHS England.

NHS National Leadership Council (2010) *The healthy NHS Board: Principles for good governance* (www.leadershipacademy.nhs.uk/wp-content/uploads/2012/11/NHSLeadership-TheHealthyNHSBoard.pdf).

Nuffield Council on Bioethics (2007) *Public health: Ethical issues*, London: Nuffield Council on Bioethics.

Office for National Statistics (2013) *Personal Well-being in the UK, 2012/13*, Statistical Bulletin, July 2013, Office for National Statistics (www.ons.gov.uk/ons/dcp171778_319478.pdf).

Oliver, A. (2009) 'Can financial incentives improve health equity?' [comment] *British Medical Journal*, vol. 339: b3847.

Oman, C.P. and Arndt, C. (2010) *Measuring governance*, Policy Briefing No. 39, Paris: OECD Development Centre.

Omaswa, F. and Boufford, J.I. (2010) *Strong ministries for strong health systems*, African Centre for Global Health and Social Transformation and New York Academy of Medicine (www.rockefellerfoundation.org/uploads/files/8819cca6-1738-4158-87fe-4d2c7b738932.pdf).

Organisation for Economic Co-operation and Development (2007) *The economics of prevention project* (www.oecd.org/health/health-systems/theeconomicsofprevention.htm).

Osmani, S. (2008) 'Participatory governance: An overview of issues and evidence', ch. 1 in *Participatory governance and the millennium development goals (MDGs)*, New York: United Nations, 1–45 (http://unpan1.un.org/intradoc/groups/public/documents/un/unpan028359.pdf).

Ottersen, O.P., Dasgupta, J., Blouin, C. et al. (2014) 'The political origins of health inequity: prospects for change', The Lancet-University of Oslo Commission on Global Governance for Health, *The Lancet*, vol. 383, pp. 63–67.

Owen, L., Morgan, A., Fischer, A., Ellis, S., Hoy, A. and Kelly, M. (2012) 'The cost-effectiveness of public health interventions', *Journal of Public Health*, vol. 34, no. 1, pp. 37–45.

Pearson, S.D. and Lieber, S.R. (2009) 'Financial penalties for the unhealthy? Ethical guidelines for holding employees responsible for their health', *Health Affairs* (Millwood) vol. 28, pp. 845–52.

Pearson, S.D., Schneider, E.C., Kleinman, K.P., Coltin, K.L. and Singer, J.A. (2008) 'The impact of pay-for-performance on health care quality in Massachusetts, 2001–2003', *Health Affairs* (Millwood), vol. 27, pp. 1167–76.

Peckham, S. and Hann, A. (2009) *Public health ethics and practice*, Bristol: The Policy Press.

Peckham, S. and Wallace, A. (2010) 'Pay for performance schemes in primary care: what have we learnt?' *Quality in Primary Care*, vol. 18, no. 2, pp. 111–16.

Perkins, N., Smith, K., Hunter, D.J., Bambra, C. and Joyce, K. (2010). '"What counts is what works"? New Labour and partnerships in public health', *Policy and Politics*, vol. 38, no. 1, pp. 101–7.

Petersen, L.A., Woodard, L.D., Urech, T., Daw, C. and Sookanan, S. (2006) 'Does pay-for-performance improve the quality of health care?' *Annals of Internal Medicine*, vol. 145, pp. 265–72.

Pickin, C., Popay, J., Staley, K., Bruce, N., Jones, C. and Gowman, N. (2002) 'Developing a model to enhance the capacity of statutory organisations to engage with lay communities', *Journal of Health Services Research and Policy*, vol. 7, no. 1, pp. 34–42.

Povall, S.L., Haigh, F.A., Abrahams, D. and Scott-Samuel, A. (2013) 'Health equity impact assessment', *Health Promotion International* doi: 10.1093/heapro/dat012.

Prime Minister's Strategy Unit (2004) *Alcohol harm reduction strategy for England*, London: Strategy Unit.

Public Health England (2013) *Longer lives* (http://longerlives.phe.org.uk/#are//par/E92000001).

Putland, C., Baum, F., Ziersch, A., Arthurson, K. and Pomagalska, D. (2013) 'Enabling pathways to health equity: developing a framework for implementing social capital in practice', *BMC Public Health*, vol. 13, p. 517.

Rhodes, R.A.W. (1996) 'The new governance: governing without government', *Political Studies*, xliv, pp. 652–67.

Rose, G. (1992) *Strategy of preventive medicine*, Oxford: Oxford University Press.

Ruta, D., Mitton, C., Bate, A. and Donaldson, C. (2005) 'Programme budgeting and marginal analysis: bridging the divide between doctors and managers', *British Medical Journal*, vol. 330, pp. 1501–3.

Saltman, R.B. (2002) 'Regulating incentives: the past and present role of the state in health care systems', *Social Science & Medicine*, vol. 54, no. 11, pp. 1677–84.

Saltman, R.B. and Ferroussier-Davis, O. (2000) 'The concept of stewardship in health policy', *Bulletin of the World Health Organisation*, vol. 78, no. 6, pp. 732–9.

Saracci, R. (2007) 'Epidemiology: a science for justice in health', *International Journal of Epidemiology*, vol. 36, pp. 265–8.

Scally, G. and Donaldson, L.J. (1998) 'Looking forward: clinical governance and the drive for quality improvement in the new NHS in England', *British Medical Journal*, vol. 317, pp. 61–5.

Scarborough, P., Bhatnagar, P., Kremlin, W.K., Allender, S., Foster, C. and Rayner, M. (2011) 'The economic burden of ill health due to diet, physical inactivity, smoking, alcohol and obesity in the UK: an update to 2006–07 NHS costs', *Journal of Public Health*, vol. 33, no. 4, pp. 527–35.

Scottish Government (2008) *Equally well: Report of the ministerial task force on health inequalities*, Edinburgh: The Scottish Government.

Secretary of State for Communities and Local Government (2006) *Strong and prosperous communities: The local government White Paper*, Cm 6939-ll, London: The Stationery Office.

Secretary of State for Communities and Local Government (2008) *Communities in control: Real people, real power*, Cm 7427, London: The Stationery Office.

Secretaries of State for Health, Wales, Scotland and Northern Ireland (1989) *Working for patients*, Cm 555, London: HMSO.

Secretary of State for Health (1997) *The new NHS: Modern, dependable*, Cm 3807, London: The Stationery Office.

Secretary of State for Health (2000) *The NHS plan: A plan for investment a plan for reform*, Cm 4818-I, London: The Stationery Office.

Secretary of State for Health (2004) *Choosing health: Making healthy choices easier*, Cm 6734, London: The Stationery Office.

Secretary of State for Health (2006) *Our health, our care, our say: A new direction for community services*, Cm 6737, London: The Stationery Office.

Secretary of State for Health (2008) *High quality care for all: NHS next stage review final report*, Cm 7432, London: The Stationery Office.

Secretary of State for Health (2009) *NHS 2010–2015: From good to great. Preventative, people-centred, productive*, Cm 7775, London: The Stationery Office.

Secretary of State for Health (2010a) *Equity and excellence: Liberating the NHS*, Cm 7881, London: The Stationery Office.

Secretary of State for Health (2010b) *Healthy lives, healthy people: Our strategy for public health in England*, Cm 7985, London: The Stationery Office.

Secretary of State for the Home Department (2012) *The government's alcohol strategy*, Cm 8336, London: The Stationery Office.

Sigfrid, L.A., Turner, C., Crook, D. and Ray, S. (2006) 'Using the UK primary care Quality and Outcomes Framework to audit health care equity: preliminary data on diabetes management', *Journal of Public Health*, vol. 28, pp. 221–5.

Smith, P. (1995) 'On the unintended consequences of publishing performance data in the public sector', *International Journal of Public Administration*, vol. 18, pp. 277–310.

Smith, P. (2013) 'Strategic targets for public services: Lessons from Canada from the English experience', The Tansley Lecture, Regina: Johnson-Shoyama Graduate School of Public Policy (www.schoolofpublicpolicy. sk.ca/_documents/_Tansley%20Lecture/2013%20/Peter%20Smith%20 Publication_web.pdf).

South, J., White, J. and Gamsu, M. (2012) *People-centred public health*, Bristol: The Policy Press.

Springett, J. (2001) 'Appropriate approaches to the evaluation of health promotion', *Critical Public Health*, vol. 11, no. 2, pp. 139–51.

Ståhl, T., Wismar, M., Ollila, E., Lahtinen, E. and Leppo, K. (eds) (2006) *Health in all policies: Prospects and potentials*, Helsinki: Finnish Ministry of Social Affairs and Health and European Observatory on Health Systems and Policies (www.euro.who.int/__data/assets/pdf_file/0003/109146/E89260.pdf).

Steel, D. and Cylus, J. (2012) 'United Kingdom (Scotland): Health system review', *Health Systems in Transition*, vol. 14, no. 9, pp. 1–150.

Storey, J., Bate, P., Buchanan, D., Green, R., Salaman, G. and Winchester, N. (2008) *New governance arrangements in the NHS: Emergent implications*, NHS/ SDO Working Paper No. 3/2008 (www.open.ac.uk/oubs/nhs-governance/ pics/d90226.pdf).

Stuckler, D. and Basu, S. (2013) *The body economic. Why austerity kills*, London: Allen Lane.

Thaler, R.H. (1994) *Quasi rational economics*, New York: Russell Sage Foundation.

Thaler, R.H. and Sunstein, C.R. (2008) *Nudge: Improving decisions about health, wealth, and happiness*, New Haven, CT: Yale University Press.

Timmins, N. (2012) *Never again? The story of the Health and Social Care Act 2012. A study in coalition government and policy making*, London: King's Fund and Institute for Government.

Townsend, A. (2005) *Multi-level governance in England: Background paper for the Office of the Deputy Prime Minister*, Durham: Durham University (https:// www.dur.ac.uk/resources/cscr/odpm/Multilevel.pdf).

Treib, O., Bahr, H. and Falkner, G. (2005) *Modes of governance: A note towards conceptual clarification*, European Governance Papers (EUROGOV) No. N-05-02.

Tuohy, A.H. (2003) 'Agency, contract, and governance: shifting shapes of accountability in the health care arena', *Journal of Health Politics, Policy and Law*, vol. 28, no. 2–3, pp. 195–215.

Tversky, A. and Kahneman, D. (1974) 'Judgement under uncertainty: heuristics and biases', *Science*, vol. 185, no. 4157, pp. 1124–31.

United Nations Development Programme (UNDP) (1997) *Governance for sustainable human development*, New York: UNDP.

UN General Assembly (1966) *International Covenant on Economic, Social and Cultural Rights. United Nations General Assembly resolution 2200A (XXI)*. Geneva: Office of the United Nations High Commissioner for Human Rights.

Verweij, M. and Dawson, A. (2007) 'The meaning of "public" in "public health"', ch. 2 in Dawson, A. and Verweij, M. (eds) *Ethics, prevention and public health*, Oxford: Oxford University Press.

Wanless, D. (2002) *Securing our future health: Taking a long term view*, Final report, London: HM Treasury.

Wanless, D. (2004) *Securing good health for the whole population*, Final report, London: HM Treasury.

Wanless, D., Appleby, J., Harrison, T. and Patel, D. (2007) *Our future health secured? A review of NHS funding and performance*, London: King's Fund.

Weale, A. (2011) 'New modes of governance, political accountability and public reason', *Government and Opposition*, vol. 46, no. 1, pp. 58–80.

Weiss, T.G. (2000) 'Governance, good governance and global governance: conceptual and actual challenges', *Third World Quarterly*, vol. 21, no. 5, pp. 795–814.

Welsh Government (2012) *Consultation to collect views about whether a public health bill is needed in Wales* (http://wales.gov.uk/consultations/healthsocialcare/publichealth/?lang=en).

White, G., Dickinson, S., Miles, N., Richardson, L., Russell, H. and Taylor, M. (2006) *Exemplars of neighbourhood governance*, London: Department for Communities and Local Government.

Whitehead, M. (1992) 'The concepts and principles of equity in health', *International Journal of Health Services*, vol. 22, pp. 429–45.

Whitehead, M. and Popay, J. (2010) 'Swimming upstream? Taking action on the social determinants of health inequalities', *Social Science & Medicine*, vol. 71, no. 7, pp. 1234–6.

WHO (World Health Organization) (1978) *Report on the International Conference on Primary Care, Alma Ata*. Geneva: WHO.

WHO (1981) *Global strategy for Health for All by the year 2000*, Geneva: WHO.

WHO (1986) *Ottawa charter for health promotion*, presented at first International Conference on Health Promotion (Ottawa, 21 November), Geneva: WHO.

WHO (2000) *World health report 2000*, Geneva: WHO.

WHO (2002) *The world health report 2002: Reducing risks, promoting healthy life*, Geneva: WHO.

WHO (2008) *Closing the gap in a generation: Health equity through action on the social determinants of health*, Commission on Social Determinants of Health Final report, Geneva: WHO.

WHO (2012a) *Health 2020: A European policy framework supporting action across government and society for health and well-being*, Copenhagen: WHO Regional Office for Europe.

WHO (2012b) *European action plan for strengthening public health capacities and services*, Copenhagen: WHO Regional Office for Europe.

WHO (2013) *Communicating the economics of social determinants of health and health inequalities*, Geneva: WHO.

Wikler, D. and Brock, D.W. (2007) 'Population bioethics. mapping a new agenda', ch. 5 in Dawson, A. and Verweij, M. (eds) *Ethics, prevention and public health*. Oxford: Oxford University Press.

Wilkinson, R.G. and Pickett, K.E. (2010) *The spirit level: Why equality is better for everyone*, London: Penguin Books.

Williams, I., Robinson, S. and Dickinson, H. (2012) *Rationing in health care: The theory and practice of priority setting*, Bristol: The Policy Press.

Williamson, O.E. (1973) 'Markets and hierarchies: some elementary considerations', *American Economic Review*, vol. 63, pp. 316–25.

Winslow, C.E.A. (1920) 'The untilled fields of public health', *Science*, vol. 51, no. 1306, pp. 23–33.

Wismar, M., Blau, J., Ernst, K. and Figueras, J. (2007) *The effectiveness of health impact assessment: Scope and limitations of supporting decision-making in Europe*, European Observatory on Health Systems and Policies, Copenhagen: World Health Organisation.

Wismar, M., McKee, M., Ernst, K., Srivastava, D. and Busse, R. (2008) *Health targets in Europe: Learning from experience*, European Observatory on Health Systems and Policies. Observatory Studies Series no. 13.

Wyatt, S. (2008) *Investing for Health project 1: The rationale and potential risks of introducing tariffs for lifestyle risk management services*, Reference group 1 paper. Birmingham: NHS West Midlands.

Yamin, A.E. (2008) 'Beyond compassion: the central role of accountability in applying a human rights framework to health', *Health and Human Rights*, vol. 10, no. 2, pp. 1–20.

Yorkshire and Humber Health Intelligence (n.d.) *Spend and outcome tool (SPOT)* (www.yhpho.org.uk/default.aspx?RID=49488).

Index

References to tables, boxes and figures are shown in *italics*

LIBRARY, UNIVERSITY OF CHESTER